Larry VandeCreek, DMin
Editor

D1523156

Professional Chaplaincy and Clinical Pastoral Education Should Become More Scientific: Yes and No

Professional Chaplaincy and Clinical Pastoral Education Should Become More Scientific: Yes and No has been co-published simultaneously as *Journal of Health Care Chaplaincy,* Volume 12, Numbers 1/2 and Volume 13, Number 1, 2002.

Pre-publication REVIEWS, COMMENTARIES, EVALUATIONS . . .

"COMPREHENSIVE. . . . A GIFT TO EVERY CHAPLAIN who seeks an in-depth understanding of the traditional fears of scientific inquiry. . . . Takes on the challenge of rethinking scientific inquiry as a possible ally improving pastoral ministry."

Rev. Ronald Nydam, PhD
Professor of Pastoral Care
Calvin Theological Seminary

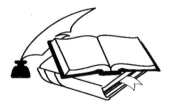

More pre-publication
REVIEWS, COMMENTARIES, EVALUATIONS . . .

"RICH AND CHALLENGING. . . . Raises important questions. . . . Makes a case for wise and thoughtful integration of science and the work of chaplains."

Homer U. Ashby, Jr., PhD
Professor of Pastoral Care
McCormick Theological Seminary

"Larry VandeCreek has rendered a singular service to clinical pastoral education and professionals chaplaincy by inviting us to become more disciplined in reflecting on the ministry of chaplains and by engaging such an intellectually stimulating dialogue. I really appreciated how this work frames accountability for effectiveness and efficiency in mediating the invisible world of presence, faith, and values. Only in this way can we who exercise a spiritual ministry ever find our place as integral members of a professional healthcare team."

Gerard T. Broccolo, STD
Vice President, Spirituality
Catholic Health Initiatives

"TIMELY . . . . MUST READING for anyone concerned about the future of chaplaincy in health care settings and about the relationship of spirituality, religion, and health."

Augustine Meier, PhD
Professor Emeritus
Clinical Psychology
Saint Paul University

"A MUST-READ for anyone trying to develop or refine a stance to support his or her specialized healthcare ministry. . . . A rich dialogue that addresses, from many perspectives, the struggle of pastoral and spiritual care in the current atmosphere of healthcare delivery."

Rev. O. Allen Lumpkin, Jr., MDiv, STM
Chair, Eastern Region, ACPE
former Director of Pastoral Care
Geisinger Medical Center

The Haworth Pastoral Press
An Imprint of The Haworth Press, Inc.

Professional Chaplaincy and Clinical Pastoral Education Should Become More Scientific: Yes and No

Professional Chaplaincy and Clinical Pastoral Education Should Become More Scientific: Yes and No has been co-published simultaneously as *Journal of Health Care Chaplaincy*, Volume 12, Numbers 1/2 and Volume 13, Number 1 2002.

The *Journal of Health Care Chaplaincy* Monographic "Separates"

Below is a list of "separates," which in serials librarianship means a special issue simultaneously published as a special journal issue or double-issue *and* as a "separate" hardbound monograph. (This is a format which we also call a "DocuSerial.")

"Separates" are published because specialized libraries or professionals may wish to purchase a specific thematic issue by itself in a format which can be separately cataloged and shelved, as opposed to purchasing the journal on an on-going basis. Faculty members may also more easily consider a "separate" for classroom adoption.

"Separates" are carefully classified separately with the major book jobbers so that the journal tie-in can be noted on new book order slips to avoid duplicate purchasing.

You may wish to visit Haworth's Website at . . .

http://www.HaworthPress.com

. . . to search our online catalog for complete tables of contents of these separates and related publications.

You may also call 1-800-HAWORTH (outside US/Canada: 607-722-5857), or Fax 1-800-895-0582 (outside US/Canada: 607-771-0012), or e-mail at:

docdelivery@haworthpress.com

Professional Chaplaincy and Clinical Pastoral Education Should Become More Scientific: Yes and No, edited by Larry VandeCreek, DMin, BCC (Vol. 12, No. 1/2, and Vol. 13, No. 1, 2002). *"Timely. . . . Must reading for anyone concerned about the future of chaplaincy in health care settings and about the relationship of spirituality, religion, and health." (Augustine Meier, PhD, Professor Emeritus, Clinical Psychology, Saint Paul University)*

The Discipline for Pastoral Care Giving: Foundations for Outcome Oriented Chaplaincy, edited by Larry VandeCreek, DMin, BCC, and Arthur M. Lucas, MDiv, BCC (Vol. 10, No. 2, 2001 and Vol. 11, No. 1, 2001). *"A cutting edge approach to spiritual care. . . . An essential resource." (George Fitchett, DMin, Associate Professor and Director of Research, Rush-Presbyterian-St. Luke's Medical Center, Chicago, Illinois)*

Professional Chaplaincy: What Is Happening to It During Health Care Reform? edited by Larry VandeCreek, DMin, BCC (Vol. 10, No. 1, 2000). *Containing firsthand accounts of the present changes in the field and suggestions for action from an Australian case study, this informative work will assist you in developing future plans for chaplaincy, ones that will take your needs into consideration and help this important job remain in care facilities.*

Contract Pastoral Care and Education: The Trend of the Future? edited by Larry VandeCreek, DMin, BCC (Vol. 9, No. 1/2, 1999). *Provides clergy of all faiths and students with information on how religious and spiritual ministries within health care benefit patients. You will discover "how to" suggestions as well as a wealth of experiences and models for planning a freestanding pastoral care center of your own to benefit your community.*

Spiritual Care for Persons with Dementia: Fundamentals for Pastoral Practice, edited by Larry VandeCreek, DMin, BCC (Vol. 8, No. 1/2, 1999). *Offers you a better understanding of dementia and how to better serve persons with this frustrating and often confusing disease.*

Scientific and Pastoral Perspectives on Intercessory Prayer: An Exchange Between Larry Dossey, MD and Health Care Chaplains, edited by Larry VandeCreek, DMin (Vol. 7, No. 1/2, 1998). *"Anyone who wonders about our prayers and our needs will be drawn into these dialogues." (Laland E. Elhard, PhD, Professor of Pastoral Theology, Trinity Lutheran Seminary, Columbus, Ohio) Summarizes Larry Dossey's work on prayer and challenges chaplains to think seriously about its role in their ministry.*

Ministry of Hospital Chaplains: Patient Satisfaction, edited by Larry VandeCreek, DMin, and Marjorie A. Lyon (Vol. 6, No. 2, 1997). *Explores patient satisfaction with the general hospital chaplain's ministry.*

Organ Transplantation in Religious, Ethical, and Social Context: No Room for Death, edited by William R. DeLong, MDiv, FCOC (Vol. 5, No. 1/2, 1993). *"I recommend this book to anyone working with transplant recipients or donor families."* (*Sharon Augustine, RN, MS, Heart and Lung Transplant Service, The Johns Hopkins Hospital, Baltimore*)

Health Care Chaplaincy in Oncology, edited by Laurel Arthur Burton, ThD, and George Handzo, MDiv (Vol. 4, No. 1/2, 1993). *"A valuable collection that speaks of the 'Modern' professional chaplain."* (*Rev. Elaine Hickman, Manager, Chaplaincy Services, Mercy General Hospital; President, The College of Chaplains, Inc.; Vice President, COMISS (Congress on Ministry in Specialized Settings)*)

The Chaplain-Physician Relationship, edited by Larry VandeCreek, DMin, and Laurel Arthur Burton, ThD (Vol. 3, No. 2, 1993). *"Recommended to both chaplains and physicians who are searching for ways to overcome the relational distance between the two professions."* (*The Journal of Pastoral Care*)

Making Chaplaincy Work: Practical Approaches, edited by Laurel Arthur Burton, ThD (Vol. 1, No. 2, 1988). *"Dr. Burton has done a first-class job of bringing together articulate writers whose content has been informed by their daily practice of ministry within healthcare settings."* (*David E. Latham, Director of Chaplaincy Services, Community United Methodist Hospital, Henderson, Kentucky*)

Published by

The Haworth Pastoral Press, 10 Alice Street, Binghamton, NY 13904-1580 USA

The Haworth Pastoral Press is an imprint of The Haworth Press, Inc., 10 Alice Street, Binghamton, NY 13904-1580 USA.

Professional Chaplaincy and Clinical Pastoral Education Should Become More Scientific: Yes and No has been co-published simultaneously as *Journal of Health Care Chaplaincy,* Volume 12, Numbers 1/2 and Volume 13, Number 1 2002.

The development, preparation, and publication of this work has been undertaken with great care. However, the publisher, employees, editors, and agents of The Haworth Press and all imprints of The Haworth Press, Inc., including The Haworth Medical Press® and The Pharmaceutical Products Press®, are not responsible for any errors contained herein or for consequences that may ensue from use of materials or information contained in this work. Opinions expressed by the author(s) are not necessarily those of The Haworth Press, Inc.

Cover design by Jennifer M. Gaska.

Library of Congress Cataloging-in-Publication Data

Professional chaplaincy and clinical pastoral education should become more scientific: yes and no / Larry VandeCreek, editor.
     p. cm.
     "Professional chaplaincy and clinical pastoral education should become more scientific: Yes and No has been co-published simultaneously as Journal of health care chaplaincy, volume 12, numbers 1/2, and Volume 13, Number 1, 2002."
     Includes bibliographical references and index.
     ISBN 0-7890-2237-0 (hard cover: alk. paper)–ISBN 0-7890-2238-9 (soft cover: alk. paper)
     1. Chaplains–Training of.   I. VandeCreek, Larry. II. Journal of health care chaplaincy
BV4375.P76 2003
253'.071'1–dc21
                                                20033011593

Professional Chaplaincy and Clinical Pastoral Education Should Become More Scientific: Yes and No

Larry VandeCreek, DMin
Editor

Professional Chaplaincy and Clinical Pastoral Education Should Become More Scientific: Yes and No has been co-published simultaneously as *Journal of Health Care Chaplaincy*, Volume 12, Numbers 1/2 and Volume 13, Number 1, 2002.

The Haworth Pastoral Press
An Imprint of The Haworth Press, Inc.
The Haworth Press, Inc.
New York

Indexing, Abstracting & Website/Internet Coverage

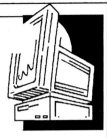

This section provides you with a list of major indexing & abstracting services. That is to say, each service began covering this periodical during the year noted in the right column. Most Websites which are listed below have indicated that they will either post, disseminate, compile, archive, cite or alert their own Website users with research-based content from this work. (This list is as current as the copyright date of this publication.)

Abstracting, Website/Indexing Coverage . . . . Year When Coverage Began

- *This periodical is indexed in ATLA Religion Database, published by the American Theological Library Association <www.atla.com>* . . . . *

- *CINAHL (Cumulative Index To Nursing & Allied Health Literature), In Print EBSCO, and SilverPlatter, Data-Star, and PaperChase. (Support materials include Subject Heading List, Database Search Guide, and instructional video). <www.cinahl.com>* 2001

- *CNPIEC Reference Guide: Chinese National Directory of Foreign Periodicals* 1995

- *Current Thoughts & Trends "Abstracts Section".* 2000

- *Family & Society Studies Worldwide <www.nisc.com>* 1995

- *Gay & Lesbian Abstracts provides comprehensive & in-depth coverage of the world's GLBT literature compiled by NISC & published on the Internet & CD-ROM <www.nisc.com>*

- *HealthSTAR* 1996

- *Help the Hospices (the National Charity for the hospice movement <www.helpthe hospice.org.uk>* 2001

- *Human Resources Abstracts (HRA)* 1990

(continued)

- *Index Guide to College Journals (core list complied by integrating 48 indexes frequently used to support undergraduate programs in small to medium sized libraries)* 1999

- *Index to Jewish Periodicals <www.jewishperiodicals.com>* . . . . *

- *Leeds Medical Information* 1996

- *MEDLINE (National Library of Medicine) (www.nlm.nih.gov)*

- *Orere Source, The (Pastoral Abstracts)* 1997

- *PubMed (National Library of Medicine) (www.nlm.nih.gov)* . . . . *

- *Religious & Theological Abstracts. For a free search and more information visit our website at: <http://www.rtabst.org>* 1998

- *Theology Digest (also made available on CD-ROM)* 1992

* *Exact start date to come.*

Special Bibliographic Notes related to special journal issues (separates) and indexing/abstracting:

- indexing/abstracting services in this list will also cover material in any "separate" that is co-published simultaneously with Haworth's special thematic journal issue or DocuSerial. Indexing/abstracting usually covers material at the article/chapter level.
- monographic co-editions are intended for either non-subscribers or libraries which intend to purchase a second copy for their circulating collections.
- monographic co-editions are reported to all jobbers/wholesalers/approval plans. The source journal is listed as the "series" to assist the prevention of duplicate purchasing in the same manner utilized for books-in-series.
- to facilitate user/access services all indexing/abstracting services are encouraged to utilize the co-indexing entry note indicated at the bottom of the first page of each article/chapter/contribution.
- this is intended to assist a library user of any reference tool (whether print, electronic, online, or CD-ROM) to locate the monographic version if the library has purchased this version but not a subscription to the source journal.
- individual articles/chapters in any Haworth publication are also available through the Haworth Document Delivery Service (HDDS).

Professional Chaplaincy and Clinical Pastoral Education Should Become More Scientific: Yes and No

CONTENTS

Preface: What Has Jerusalem to Do with Athens? What Has
Pastoral Care to Do with Science?   xiii

Chaplain No: Should Clinical Pastoral Education
and Professional Chaplaincy Become More Scientific
in Response to Health Care Reform?   xv

Chaplain Yes: Should Clinical Pastoral Education
and Professional Chaplaincy Become More Scientific
in Response to Health Care Reform?   xvii

Should Clinical Pastoral Education and Professional Chaplaincy
Become More Scientific?
It's a Matter of Salt   1
Joe Baroody, DMin, BCC

Spirituality and Data: The Need for a New Paradigm   11
Rev. William J. Baugh, DMin, BCC

To Be, Or Not To Be More Scientific? That Is the Question:
Yes, Absolutely, But . . .   19
Paul Steven Bay, DMin, BCC

Chaplains and Science   29
W. Noel Brown, STM, BCC

Chaplaincy *Is* Becoming More "Scientific." What's
the Problem?   43
    Larry Burton, ThD, BCC

Clinical Pastoral Education and the Value of Empirical Research:
Examples from Australian and New Zealand Datum   53
    Rev. Chap. Lindsay B. Carey, MAppSc, RAAF
    Rev. Dr. Christopher Newell, AM, PhD

Health Care Chaplaincy as a Research-Informed Profession:
How We Get There   67
    George Fitchett, DMin, BCC

Science and Ministry: Confusion and Reality   73
    The Rev. George F. Handzo, MDiv, BCC

Siblings or Foes: What Now in Spiritual Care Research?   81
    Gordon J. Hilsman, DMin, BCC

Research or Perish?   91
    Margot Hover, DMin

Ministry for the Good of the Whole   99
    Eugene W. Huffstutler, DMin, BCC

Chaplain Yes and Chaplain No: Both Are Correct;
Neither Is True   103
    Steven S. Ivy, PhD

Language and Tools for Professional Accountability   113
    Mark E. Jensen, PhD

Four Fatal Flaws in Recent Spirituality Research   125
    Raymond J. Lawrence, DMin

In the World but Not of the World: Going Beyond a Dilemma   131
    Richard Leliaert, OSC, PhD

At the Poles Eventually All You Get Is Cold   143
    Chaplain Arthur M. Lucas, MDiv, BCC

But What Are We Trying to Prove?   151
    David B. McCurdy, DMin, BCC

She Said, "Some Patient Needs Get Dropped Due
    to More Pressing Issues"   165
    Dick Millspaugh, MDiv, BCC

Respecting the Dual Sided Identity
    of Clinical Pastoral Education and Professional Chaplaincy:
    The Phenomenological Research Model   171
    Marie-Line Morin, PhD

The Search for Truth: The Case for Evidence Based Chaplaincy   185
    Thomas St. James O'Connor, ThD

Health Care Reform: Opportunities for Professional Chaplains
    to Build Intentional Communities of Learners by Integrating
    Faith, Science, Quality, and Systems Thinking   195
    Bartholomew Rodrigues, MDiv, MA, BCC

The Chaplain as the Complete Philosopher   213
    Orlo C. Strunk, Jr., PhD

Rediscovering Mystery and Wonder:
    Toward a Narrative-Based Perspective on Chaplaincy   223
    Rev. Dr. John Swinton, PhD, BD, RMN, RNMH

Attention to the Scientific Benefits of Pastoral Care Is a Blessing
    and a Curse   237
    The Reverend Jo Clare Wilson, MDiv

Index   245

ABOUT THE EDITOR

Larry VandeCreek, DMin, BCC, is Director of Pastoral Research at The HealthCare Chaplaincy in New York City. For 23 years, he held faculty and staff positions with The Ohio State University College of Medicine and Public Health and its associated medical center. Dr. VandeCreek is a member of numerous professional associations including the Association of Professional Chaplains, Inc., the American Association of Pastoral Counselors, and the Association for Clinical Pastoral Education. He has published many journal articles which examine aspects of the relationship between religious faith and illness. Dr. VandeCreek is the author of *A Research Primer for Pastoral Care and Counseling* (Journal of Pastoral Care Publications, 1988) and is Co-Editor of *The Chaplain-Physician Relationship* (1991). He is Editor of the *Journal of Health Care Chaplaincy* (The Haworth Press, Inc.) which has published *Ministry of Hospital Chaplains: Patient Satisfaction* (1997), *Scientific and Pastoral Perspectives on Intercessory Prayer: An Exchange Between Larry Dossey, M.D. and Health Care Chaplains* (1998), *Spiritual Care for Persons with Dementia: Fundamentals for Pastoral Practice* (1999), *Contract Pastoral Care and Education: The Trend of the Future?* (1999), *Professional Chaplaincy: What Is Happening to It During Health Care Reform?* (2000), and *The Discipline for Pastoral Care Giving: Foundations for Outcome Oriented Chaplaincy* (2001).

Preface:
What Has Jerusalem to Do with Athens?
What Has Pastoral Care
to Do with Science?

Perhaps the question about this relationship first arose when the early church asked whether their religious faith could in some way be joined with Greek philosophy or Roman rhetoric. Tertullian gave one answer: "What indeed has Jerusalem to do with Athens? What concord is there between the Academy and the Church?" (Lischer, 2002). The answer was clear: Nothing! Augustine gave another answer–and a definitive one for a long time. He adapted Cicero, replying to Tertullian, in effect, "Why do pagans get to brandish their persuasive artillery while Christians stand by tongue-tied and unarmed?" (Lischer, 2002).

But the question of the relationship of the secular and the religious could not easily be put to rest. It came up over and over in various forms. It emerged as a major concern when the church struggled with Galileo and Copernicus: Doesn't science corrupt theology? The question today, at least in pastoral care circles, is "What has pastoral care to do with science?" This is a very practical question concerning whether and what scientific methods are appropriate. Should pastoral care and counseling become more scientific in their methodologies?

The field of pastoral counseling has faced a similar question and clearly answered "yes." Pastoral counseling makes extensive use of the sciences of psychological testing and psychotherapeutic skills–all the products of scientific thinking.

[Haworth indexing entry note]: "Preface: What Has Jerusalem to Do with Athens? What has Pastoral Care to Do with Science?" VandeCreek, Larry. Published in *Professional Chaplaincy and Clinical Pastoral Education Should Become More Scientific: Yes and No* (ed: Larry VandeCreek) The Haworth Pastoral Press, an imprint of The Haworth Press, Inc., 2003, pp. xiii-xiv. Single or multiple copies of this article are available for a fee from The Haworth Document Delivery Service [1-800-HAWORTH, 9:00 a.m. - 5:00 p.m. (EST). E-mail address: docdelivery@haworthpress.com].

The field of pastoral care has answered "yes." The thinking of behavioral scientists heavily influences its clinical education and practice, (e.g., Carl Rogers; Sigmund Freud). Augustine would likely be proud.

So is it even necessary to raise the question discussed in this volume: "Should chaplaincy become more scientific?" Given the history sketched above–howbeit all too briefly–one would think not. Chaplaincy already is scientific. And yet discussion seems necessary because widespread ambivalence exists.

The materials here were created by simply inviting authors to respond to two short pieces that appear at the beginning of this volume. Titled "Chaplain No" and "Chaplain Yes," they briefly state their position regarding this question. I then invited a wide variety of persons in pastoral care and counseling to respond. I made no effort to influence the more than 20 responses I received.

Some authors take a historical perspective. Others give voice to their additional questions and concerns. A few make concrete proposals as to how chaplaincy can become more scientific. Hopefully this volume will generate additional discussion and contribute to clearer perspectives about whether and how chaplaincy should become more scientific.

My efforts to arrange the responses into categories failed. I simply use the author's last name to present them here in alphabetical order.

Larry VandeCreek, DMin, BCC

REFERENCE

Lischer, R. (Aug. 26-September 10, 2002). Making preaching come alive: Repeat performance. *Christian Century* 119(18), 22-25.

Chaplain No:
Should Clinical Pastoral Education and Professional Chaplaincy Become More Scientific in Response to Health Care Reform?

NO! THEY WILL LOSE THEIR VOICE JUST WHEN THEY NEED IT MOST

Clinical pastoral education and health care chaplaincy need to pray, "Lead us not into temptation!" That prayer may help them resist health care reform pressures sorely tempting them to become scientific disciplines. If they give in to the temptation, they will become minor scientifically oriented professionals in the eyes of all concerned–and those in need of spiritual care don't need scientific professionals. Clinical pastoral education and chaplaincy, like all of ministry, is an art and not a science. They have a more significant calling than to be scientific; it is to represent the love of the Transcendent during illness, despair, and death. They will not be able to carry out that mission as scientific disciplines because science will also define them, shaping them into siblings of allied health disciplines. Now that corporate values have taken over health care delivery, clinical pastoral education and chaplaincy need to speak more clearly than ever before from outside science and its methods. And just when their voice must be most clear, they are tempted to sell out to the business and scientific ethic by trying to reduce ministry to numbers. Some believe they can justify their ministry by statistically

[Haworth co-indexing entry note]: "Chaplain No: Should Clinical Pastoral Education and Professional Chaplaincy Become More Scientific In Response to Health Care Reform?." VandeCreek, Larry. Co-published simultaneously in *Journal of Health Care Chaplaincy* (The Haworth Pastoral Press, an imprint of The Haworth Press, Inc.) Vol. 12, No. 1/2, 2003, pp. xix-xv; and: *Professional Chaplaincy and Clinical Pastoral Education Should Become More Scientific: Yes and No* (ed: Larry VandeCreek) The Haworth Pastoral Press, an imprint of The Haworth Press, Inc., 2003, pp. xv-xvi. Single or multiple copies of this article are available for a fee from The Haworth Document Delivery Service [1-800-HAWORTH, 9:00 a.m. - 5:00 p.m. (EST). E-mail address: docdelivery@haworthpress.com].

demonstrating its outcomes, thereby hoping to convince scientists and administrators that their services are necessary and important. I argue that such an attempt to sell chaplaincy cannot be accomplished without selling out the very essence of ministry. Clinical pastoral education and chaplaincy are morally obligated to resist this seduction by science and health care reform.

Larry VandeCreek, DMin, BCC

Chaplain Yes:
Should Clinical Pastoral Education
and Professional Chaplaincy
Become More Scientific in Response
to Health Care Reform?

YES! THEY WILL FIND THEIR VOICE
JUST WHEN THEY NEED IT MOST

Clinical pastoral education and health care chaplaincy need to pray, "Lead us not into temptation!" Health care reform offers a significant opportunity to improve ministry by using scientific tools although clinical pastoral education and professional chaplaincy are tempted to ignore the opportunity. As technology becomes more dominant and business perspectives manage health care, clinical pastoral education and chaplaincy are called to support those experiencing illness, despair, and death by presenting the message of the great religious traditions. They cannot expect to do that by holding themselves aloof, outside the circle of other professionals who seek to help. Yet, just when their voice must be most clear, they are tempted to sell out once again to the old self-proclaimed assertions that they are helpful and that no scientific investigation is necessary–the very assertions that seem so questionable to scientists and administrative decision makers. While clinical pastoral education and chaplaincy intuitively know that they are helpful, they need to use scientific methods to demonstrate it. The results will strengthen their ministry, suggesting ways in which this ministry can be even more effective. Such results will be convincing to decision-makers

---

[Haworth co-indexing entry note]: "Chaplain Yes: Should Clinical Pastoral Education and Professional Chaplaincy Become More Scientific in Response to Health Care Reform?" VandeCreek, Larry. Co-published simultaneously in *Journal of Health Care Chaplaincy* (The Haworth Pastoral Press, an imprint of The Haworth Press, Inc.) Vol. 13, No. 1/2, 2002, pp. xxi-xxii; and: *Professional Chaplaincy and Clinical Pastoral Education Should Become More Scientific: Yes and No* (ed: Larry VandeCreek) The Haworth Pastoral Press, an imprint of The Haworth Press, Inc., 2002, pp. xvii-xviii. Single or multiple copies of this article are available for a fee from The Haworth Document Delivery Service [1-800-HAWORTH, 9:00 a.m. - 5:00 p.m. (EST). E-mail address: docdelivery@haworthpress.com].

http://www.haworthpress.com/store/product.asp?sku=J080
xvii

who will then more clearly understand why ministry is necessary and how it is helpful. Science and health care reform can be very helpful to clinical pastoral education and chaplaincy and I argue that they are morally obligated to use scientific methods to measure the helpfulness of their practices and to improve them. If they do not do so, they will continue to imply that they are above the scrutiny required of their peer health care professionals.

Larry VandeCreek, DMin, BCC

Should Clinical Pastoral Education and Professional Chaplaincy Become More Scientific? It's a Matter of Salt

Joe Baroody, DMin, BCC

SUMMARY. I address the relationship of Clinical Pastoral Education (CPE) and professional chaplaincy to science by looking at the past in order to find meaning for the present. Specially, I explore the stories of Elwood Worcester, Anton Boisen and the beginnings of CPE. I conclude that these and other founding fathers believed that they were called to continue Christ's healing ministry and turned to science as a means to do so although their relationship to science was often strained. Three issues emerge from the past that offer meaning for the present: the significance of a spiritual calling to do healing, the significance of science's "salt effect" as the means that makes a healing ministry possible, and the significance of faith as the identity around which a relationship with science is developed. *[Article copies available for a fee from The Haworth Document Delivery Service: 1-800-HAWORTH. E-mail address: <docdelivery@haworthpress.com> Website: <http://www.HaworthPress.com> © 2002 by The Haworth Press, Inc. All rights reserved.]*

Joe Baroody is affiliated with the Baroody Pastoral Counseling Center, 252 South Dargan Street, Florence, SC 29506 (E-mail: Blakelybaroody@aol.com).

[Haworth co-indexing entry note]: "Should Clinical Pastoral Education and Professional Chaplaincy Become More Scientific? It's A Matter of Salt." Baroody, Joe. Co-published simultaneously in *Journal of Health Care Chaplaincy* (The Haworth Pastoral Press, an imprint of The Haworth Press, Inc.) Vol. 12, No. 1/2, 2002, pp. 1-10; and: *Professional Chaplaincy and Clinical Pastoral Education Should Become More Scientific: Yes and No* (ed: Larry VandeCreek) The Haworth Pastoral Press, an imprint of The Haworth Press, Inc., 2003, pp. 1-10. Single or multiple copies of this article are available for a fee from The Haworth Document Delivery Service [1-800-HAWORTH, 9:00 a.m. - 5:00 p.m. (EST). E-mail address: docdelivery@haworthpress.com].

http://www.haworthpress.com/store/product.asp?sku=J080
10.1300/J080v12n01_01

KEYWORDS. Chaplaincy, pastoral care, science, clinical pastoral education

INTRODUCTION

In her 1985 book, *Ministry After Freud*, Allison Stokes reminds us, "How we interpret the past will determine the meaning we find in the present and the action we take in the future" (p. xiii). Thus, before considering the question, "Should clinical pastoral education (CPE) and professional chaplaincy become more scientific in response to health care reform?" these organizations would do well to investigate the past. Insights gained from the past would reveal that before Chaplain Yes and Chaplain No pray "Lead us not into temptation," they should first meditate upon Matthew 5:13, "You are the salt of the earth." This salt metaphor, which refers to its taste and preservation, best captures the history of these relationships. While problems have always existed between science and these two organizations, historically, science has been the salt that has flavored and preserved the health care role of CPE and professional chaplaincy. Stokes wonderfully demonstrates this by telling the stories of the religion and health pioneers.

For my purposes here, I focus on the stories of Elwood Worcester who began the Emmanuel Movement, Anton Boisen who was the father of CPE, and the beginning of the CPE Movement. The origins, accomplishments, and problems of a partnership that began early in the twentieth century, offers insight into the type of partnership CPE and professional chaplaincy can have with science as the twenty-first century begins.

I draw three conclusions from Stokes' (1985) materials. First, Worcester, Boisen, and early CPE leaders such as Flanders Dunbar and Seward Hiltner strongly believed that they were called to continue Christ's healing ministry. Theirs was more than a calling to support people experiencing illness, despair and death as Chaplain Yes states. It also took on more significance than simply representing the love of the Transcendent as Chaplain No claims. They were called, in the name of Christ, to be healers. Second, through collaboration with psychological and medical science, in which science salted the insights of theology, a new method of healing was created and developed. Third, the "salt effect" of science, however, created a tense, often strained partnership leading to disputes both between science and these movements and within the movements themselves. Yet, despite the problems or perhaps because of them, these movements can be said to have reformed health care in the twentieth century.

A LOOK AT THE PAST

In 1906, the Rev. Dr. Elwood Worcester organized the Emmanuel Movement. As rector of Emmanuel Church, Boston's largest Episcopal congregation, he became concerned that the institutional church no longer influenced people's lives. The impersonal nature of the Social Gospel and society's attraction to the healing claims of Christian Science greatly distressed him. To recover Christ's healing ministry, Worcester turned to real science. Stokes states, "Scientific psychotherapy became the means for God's cure of souls . . ." (p. 30). This healing method distinguished itself from faith healing, which relied on Biblical literalism, by combining "the insights of faith and science" (p. 31).

To employ scientific psychotherapy as a means of recovering Christ's healing ministry, Worcester turned to medical science for help. He and his assistant, the Rev. Dr. Samuel McComb, united with Boston physicians James Jackson Putnam, Richard Cabot and Isador Coriat. Without their support, says Stokes (1985), "the work would not have proceeded" · (p. 29). Besides teaching them the value of keeping confidential records, these physicians rendered a medical diagnosis that let Worcester and McComb know if their treatment could be effective.

Not everybody applauded this collaboration with science. According to Stokes, the Rev. George B. Cutten of Yale Divinity School believed that clergy who took up therapeutic work were of no use to the church. Such work only compromised the minister's role of morally and spiritually developing humanity. As it turned out, Dr. Putnam also agreed. He accused Worcester and McComb of leading a new medical movement. To resolve this problem he called for clergy-physician roles to be clarified. Nonetheless, this new form of healing ministry lasted until 1929 when Worcester resigned the church. During his tenure at Emmanuel, Worcester helped a middle-aged minister named Anton Boisen who was in love with a woman who did not return his affections.

Boisen's story parallels that of Worcester. He too felt called to a healing ministry, relying on both psychological and medical science as a means for practicing this ministry and experiencing conflict with medical science over boundary issues. Just as the combination of theology and science in Worcester's ministry launched the Emmanuel Movement, the same combination in Boisen's ministry launched the CPE movement.

Boisen's journey begins at age forty-three when he had a psychotic episode as a result of his failed love affair with Alice Batchelder. This, and subsequent episodes, kept him hospitalized from October 1920 until January 1922. Within two weeks, the initial psychosis was over and Boisen began searching for ways to understand what had happened to him. He found little guidance from his medical doctors who told him his mental illness stemmed from some mysterious organic problem (Stokes, 1985, 40). Frustrated with this explanation, he turned to a friend, the Rev. Fred Eastman, who introduced him to the new ideas of Freud. As an "evangelical liberal," Boisen believed his psychosis had an underlying spiritual purpose. It was not simply an organic problem. Freud's concepts of the unconscious and transference gave Boisen the understanding and peace he sought. He realized that in order to find healing he needed to resolve his transference to Alice. With Eastman's help, he made plans to undergo psychoanalysis at another hospital. Another relapse, however, prevented his transfer. Eventually, Boisen received help from Dr. Elwood Worcester.

During the time between his relapse and his treatment from Dr. Worcester, Boisen discovered that his true calling was a ministry to the mentally ill. After his release from the hospital, he returned to seminary to study the problems of mental illness. Stokes says Boisen came to accept what he termed "dynamic thinking" (p. 45) which "views mental life as the interplay of reciprocally urging and checking forces" (p. xvii). Freud's theories confirmed for him the validity of this way of understanding mental illness. The significance of this is that the combination of Boisen's evangelical faith and Freudian theory resulted in a new method of healing, one even different from Worcester who did not turn to Freud until later in life. Just to be clear, Freud's dynamic psychology was considered to be scientifically valid, not only by Boisen and Worcester, but also by other religious and health leaders such as Dunbar, Blanton, Hiltner and Tillich.

Like Worcester, Boisen depended upon the medical community and medical science, particularly Dr. Richard Cabot. As he did with Worcester, Cabot also taught Boisen the value of case presentation. Boisen later used this concept to develop the case method in theological education. In 1924, Cabot also recommended Boisen to Dr. William A. Bryan for the position of chaplain at Worcester State Hospital in Massachusetts. There, Boisen became interested in offering clinical training for theological students. Again Cabot helped. His article, "A Plea for a Clinical

Year in the Course of Theological Study," strongly influenced the beginning of the CPE movement. Thus, in June 1925, Boisen began a clinical training program at Worcester State Hospital. Without Cabot's help none of this would have been possible; yet, Boisen and Cabot eventually parted ways.

Strong differences over the origins of mental illness caused the two of them to sever ties. Cabot supported the organic explanation for mental illness, believing there was a chemistry to depression. As a result, Cabot sought to restrict the chaplain's role solely to the comfort and support of the mentally ill. Boisen was convinced of the psychological, spiritual explanation and so advocated a more direct role for the chaplain in the healing process. Their differences culminated in November 1930, when Cabot withdrew his support of the training program at Worcester. In 1932, Boisen left Worcester and organized a training program at Elgin State Hospital near Chicago. He remained there until his death in 1965.

With the direct connection between Worcester, Boisen and the clinical training of theological students, it should come as no surprise that the same issues of calling, partnership with science and ensuing conflict, continued as the CPE movement developed. By 1929, Boisen's training program had grown to fifteen students. In January 1930, the program became officially known as the Council for Clinical Training of Theological Students, and its focus was to continue Boisen's mission of a healing ministry. Stokes (1985) quotes professor Edward Thornton as he describes the rise of clinical pastoral education: "Clinical pastoral education may be said to be an effort by the religious community to secure the fires of healing for the altars of the church and synagogue" (p. 66).

Once again, a partnership with medical science enabled the Council to survive. Helen Flanders Dunbar, MD, one of Boisen's original students, became the Council's medical director. The residence of Dr. Cabot was designated as the official headquarters. And once again, dissension broke out. The Council's field secretary, Philip Guiles, another early student of Boisen's, clashed with Dunbar, splitting the Council in 1932 into the Boston group and the New York group. Stokes (1985) points out that the two groups continued the Cabot-Boisen controversy over the origins of mental illness and the role of the chaplain. The Boston group, led by Guiles, associated with Cabot, while the New York group, headed by Dunbar, sided with Boisen. Despite this split, it is noteworthy that Cabot and Dunbar, two medical doctors, who despite their differences, had a major impact in continuing this movement which, in 1967, became the Association for Clinical Pastoral Education.

This love-hate relationship with science has continued throughout the history of CPE. Philosopher Jenny Yates Hammett (1975) referring to the late 1930s-early 1940s split between Seward Hiltner (of the Boisen-Dunbar tradition) and Robert E. Brinkman (Cabot tradition), states that CPE "appears not to have changed its basic liberal orientation of scientific method over theological content" (p. 88-89). Her call for a renewed focus on theology was met by Henri Nouwen's address on spirituality at the 1976 ACPE conference in Detroit. ACPE historian, John Thomas (2000) states that since then some CPE centers have developed seminars on theology/spirituality as a part of their curriculum.

This look at the past reminds us that from their early roots CPE and professional chaplaincy have needed science. Science made the spiritual calling to a healing ministry a reality. Through science, religion created a viable, practical and reliable method of healing. Despite all the problems, this partnership changed health care in the twentieth century. Thomas (2000) states that CPE in the last 75 years "has changed the health and welfare institutions of the United States . . ." (p. 108). He notes that CPE influenced the Hospice Movement, contributed to the rise of ecumenism, supported the training of lay ministers, and helped develop the Parish Nurse program.

What will happen in the next 75 years? I suggest that there are three issues that guided Worcester, Boisen and the pioneers of the CPE. These same three issues can also play an important role in helping CPE and professional chaplaincy make decisions regarding their relationship with science in the twenty-first century. The issues are: (1) The significance of their spiritual calling–Worcester and Boisen felt called to continue Jesus' priestly, healing ministry. Their collaboration with science created a new method of healing. (2) The significance of science's "salt effect" on their healing ministry–the collaboration with science made it possible to practice the ministry of healing. (3) The significance of faith–Worcester and Boisen were firmly grounded in an evangelical, liberal faith. Science simply affirmed an identity that already existed. I now explore how these issues affect the current question: Should CPE and professional chaplaincy become more scientific in response to health care reform?

MEANING FOR THE PRESENT

CPE and professional chaplaincy cannot address this question without first addressing the significance of their calling. Both Chaplain Yes and Chaplain No refer to this calling as being supportive to the sick by "presenting the message of the great religious traditions" and representing "the love of the Transcendent." These authors then argue whether or not science should be used as a means to justify this calling to decision-makers. Such justification is of little value, however, if CPE and professional chaplaincy are vague about, or even ignorant of, what they are specifically called to do.

One thing is certain: Worcester and Boisen were clear about the nature of their calling and they fought quite hard to defend it. Worcester and Boisen were called to be healers. Representing God's love and being supportive to the sick were aspects of their calling but by no means did these roles define it. Neither Chaplain Yes nor Chaplain No even mention healing in their reference to calling. The distinction between being a healer in the name of God and being supportive in the name of God was crucial then and remains crucial today.

For Worcester and Boisen, the call to be healers meant continuing the priestly, healing ministry of Jesus. They were called to actually bring "healing–understood as wholeness, integration, or "salvation"–to hurting people (Stokes, 1985, p. 161)." This meant they viewed humans as Jesus did–a unity of body, mind and spirit. More than anything else, this meant creating a new method of healing by applying the principles of science. Until this time, unless it was the faith healing of Biblical literalism, the primary tools clergy used were intuitive gifts and life experience. Unfortunately, these tools limited the healing ministry to a supportive role. Worcester and Boisen wanted to move beyond this to a more active role that had a direct therapeutic effect.

This distinction took on further importance when they met resistance from Richard Cabot who fought to keep clergy in a supportive role, answering to medical doctors. Cabot (1936) makes his position clear in *The Art of Ministering To The Sick*, a book co-authored with Rev. Russell L. Dicks. In a chapter he wrote, Cabot offers "hints" on the clergy-doctor roles. The second hint reads, "By the patient's or the family's mandate the doctor is as much the boss in illness as the minister is at the funeral. The doctor rightly does not want interference with his job or question of his authority within his field" (p. 51). The sixth hint reads: "Don't practice psychotherapy in any technical sense (or so that the patient or doctor know it). Come as a friend or as a minister and not as a healer; then you will get on well with the doctors" (p. 51).

What enabled Worcester and Boisen to follow through with their healing ministry, despite the resistance of decision-makers like Cabot, was the clarity of their calling and the fierceness of their commitment. Thus, before arguing about using science to justify their ministry, CPE and professional chaplaincy should be clear about their calling as healers who first utilize science as a means to do this ministry. Before they can fight to do it, they must know what they are called to do.

Utilizing science as the means for continuing the priestly, healing ministry of Jesus brings us to the second issue: science's "salt effect" on this healing ministry. When Worcester and Boisen turned to science as the means for implementing a new method of healing, what did science actually do that made it a healing, as opposed to a supportive, ministry? It's simple. In the same way the flavor of salt gives new life to bland food, the flavor of science gave new life to pastoral ministry. Science literally turned pastoral care and counseling into a healing ministry. Stokes says scientific psychology, particularly the concepts of Freud, revealed the laws of mental health. This discovery answered "the need for confidence and competence in pastoral care and counseling without which ministry was threatened with becoming irrelevant in America" (Stokes, 1985, p. 159). Science further exhibited salt's preserving quality by making pastoral care and counseling teachable disciplines giving clergy the necessary tools to understand themselves and others with greater clarity. Thus, the salt of science gave pastoral care and counseling a "measure of mastery" that brought healing to overwhelmed Americans in the "fractured fragmented time" (Stokes, 1985, 160-161) that characterized America at the turn of the twentieth century.

The recent bombing of the World Trade Center illustrates how the term "fractured and fragmented" also characterizes America now, at the turn of the twenty-first century. As organizations that specialize in the teaching and practicing of pastoral care and counseling, CPE and professional chaplaincy cannot afford to see themselves as an art that does not need the salt of science if they wish to speak to the needs of overwhelmed Americans today. Attempts to do so would doom them to irrelevancy and oblivion.

While history reminds us of science's invaluable role to the healing ministry of CPE and professional chaplaincy, it also attests to the divisions caused by science's salt effect. The conflicts of Putnam-Worcester, Cabot-Boisen, Guiles-Dunbar and Brinkman-Hiltner all dealt with whether the sacred was being sacrificed for the secular. This same issue presents CPE and professional chaplaincy with their greatest challenge: that of maintaining their faith identity when science tempts them with its own version of faith. Stokes emphasizes that religion and health leaders like Worcester and Boisen avoided the temptation of tipping the scales toward the secular because they were firmly grounded in their evangelical liberal faith, "and were not persons to flit from one passing theological or psychological fad to another in search of an elusive identity or security" (p. 149).

The theological fads that currently tempt CPE and professional chaplaincy are the scientific studies claiming that faith leads to better health. They create an illusion by presenting empirical evidence that only associates religious activity and beliefs with improved health. The researcher then leaps to the theological conclusion that such evidence means that faith heals. The claim is misleading because, as James Fowler (1990) carefully points out, "faith needs to be distinguished from religion and from belief or believing . . . faith is more than intellectual assent to propositions of dubious verifiability . . ." (p. 394).

When pastoral care departments uncritically accept such studies and then use them to justify their ministries to administrators, they are sacrificing their faith identity for an identity provided by science. Evidence that professional chaplaincy has been yielding to this temptation was demonstrated by the fact that Dr. Harold Koenig was chosen as a plenary speaker at the 2000 Annual Conference of the Association of Professional Chaplains (APC) and the National Association of Catholic Chaplains (NACC). Dr. Koenig is Associate Professor of Psychiatry and Director of the Center for the Study of Religion/Spirituality and Health at Duke University Medical Center.

Dr. Koenig's (1999) article, "The Healing Power of Faith," (which originally appeared in the *Annals of Long-Term Care*) was included among the conference workshop papers published by the APC and NACC. The article begins: "Health professionals are beginning to appreciate seriously the role that religious faith plays in the lives of older people . . ." (p. 381). Faith, religious or otherwise, is rarely seen in this article. This role of religious faith is actually about how "Religious beliefs and practices become particularly important to older persons when they become sick" (p. 381). Throughout the article Dr. Koenig cites studies that support the significance of religion, not faith, in coping with illness.

Accepting the so-called scientific faith claims of medical researchers like Dr. Koenig may help professional chaplaincy survive health care reform, but in doing so, they will have traded the evangelical, liberal faith proclaimed by Elwood Worcester and Anton Boisen for an identity based on the pseudo-faith created by science.

CONCLUSION

CPE and professional chaplaincy will always need science's salt effect. Their relationship with science will probably always remain tense. At its best, the tension both flavors and preserves the healing ministry. This ministry should be guided by a spiritual call to do healing, by reaching out to science as a means to fulfill that calling, and by maintaining a faith identity that science enhances.

Using these guidelines may not always convince the decision-makers, but as Stokes (1985) concludes, they share a common belief in the healing power of truth. Speaking of truth, I remember well a statement by a CPE supervisor who said, "The truth may set you free but it won't always feel good."

REFERENCES

Cabot, Richard C. & Dicks, Russell L. (1936). *The Art of Ministering to the Sick.* New York: The Macmillan Company.

Fowler, J. W. (1990). Faith/Belief. In: *The Dictionary of Pastoral Care and Counseling.* Nashville: Abingdon Press, 394-397.

Hammett, Jenny Y. (1975). A second drink at the well: Theological and philosophical context of CPE origins. *The Journal of Pastoral Care,* 29(2), 86-89.

Koenig, Harold G. (1999). The healing power of faith. *Annals of Long-Term Care,* 7(10), 381-384.

Stokes, Allison. (1985). *Ministry After Freud.* New York: The Pilgrims Press.

Thomas, John R. (2000). *A "Snap Shot" History (1975-2000) of the Association for Clinical Pastoral Education, Inc.: A Celebration of the 75th Anniversary of CPE.* Decatur, GA: Association for Clinical Pastoral Education.

Spirituality and Data:
The Need
for a New Paradigm

Rev. William J. Baugh, DMin, BCC

SUMMARY. My ministry has meaning for me, and I trust, for others whom I serve. In times past, that meaning was sufficient testimony regarding its significance. Today, however, more scientific evidence seems needed–although I resist it and am skeptical that in the end science can really help us. Yet, the task we face, the central question facing the profession is, "Are there true, definable outcomes that can be validated when our primary task is dealing with matters of the heart and soul?" *[Article copies available for a fee from The Haworth Document Delivery Service: 1-800-HAWORTH. E-mail address: <docdelivery@haworthpress.com> Website: <http://www.HaworthPress.com> © 2002 by The Haworth Press, Inc. All rights reserved.]*

KEYWORDS. Chaplaincy, pastoral care, science

Rev. William J. Baugh is affiliated with Tampa General Hospital, Tampa, FL (E-mail: wbaugh@tgh.org).

[Haworth co-indexing entry note]: "Spirituality and Data: The Need for a New Paradigm." Baugh, William J. Co-published simultaneously in *Journal of Health Care Chaplaincy* (The Haworth Pastoral Press, an imprint of The Haworth Press, Inc.) Vol. 12, No. 1/2, 2002, pp. 11-17; and: *Professional Chaplaincy and Clinical Pastoral Education Should Become More Scientific: Yes and No* (ed: Larry VandeCreek) The Haworth Pastoral Press, an imprint of The Haworth Press, Inc., 2003, pp. 11-17. Single or multiple copies of this article are available for a fee from The Haworth Document Delivery Service [1-800-HAWORTH, 9:00 a.m. - 5:00 p.m. (EST). E-mail address: docdelivery@haworthpress.com].

10.1300/J080v12n01_02

HOW I HAVE RESISTED THIS DAY!
I HAVE WISHED THAT IT WOULD NEVER COME!

I have yearned for the good old days when holding a hand was an expression of my desire to care, my commitment to ministry and not a means to reduce the length of stay. My development as a professional chaplain involved learning how to assess the impact of my involvement and I came to believe deeply that my ministrations were helpful. I knew they were important to me but I often knew that I had made a big difference in the patient's care, that my presence was important to the person, to the family, and hopefully, to God.

I remember as though it were yesterday how moved I was that day in my first unit of CPE when a woman with end stage renal disease took her last loud breath and died right as I ended a prayer with her family. What an incredible experience! Those of us in chaplaincy know the experience well–so very sad, yet so terribly exhilarating. What an incredible privilege to be a part of that sacred experience. That event validated the importance of my work with the patient and family like no money, no authority, no plaudits ever could. Providing a pastoral presence to care deeply was what ministry was all about. I knew this was what I wanted to choose as my career and also what I wanted to teach so that others could experience a similar fullness of purpose and vocational clarity. That my ministry was important to the family was not a question. They stated it unequivocally. I knew they and I would remember this moment for the rest of our lives. The name of that woman has been long lost to memory, but the profound effect she had on my life will live as long as I do.

But what meaning did my ministry to her and her family have beyond those of us involved and, in the end, does it really matter? For example, what difference did this event, so sacred to those of us involved, make to hospital administration about the need for chaplaincy services? What effect, what benefit, if any, did it have on hospital finances? How does one scientifically prove the meaning and benefit of, the effect of all of this for the patient's family? The staff members? What real difference did my presence and prayer make to the length of stay, to the cost of her care? How does one prove that the way that we agonize with those who have lost loved ones saves the hospital money because they are less likely to sue? We who do it day by day know that it does. We can point to encounters and experiences where it clearly is so. But, how can we effectively study this issue and factor out contingencies that will assure that our conclusions are valid? This is not an easy task in the soft science of pastoral care. All of the above are related to what today is called "outcomes."

We all know of courageous attempts to conduct such studies. All of the studies have been criticized by at least a few other researchers. In fact, research methodologies are as easy to criticize as verbatim reports. I am not an historian of these studies but I remember the excitement I felt when Dr. Elizabeth McSherry's 1986 study came out. You will remember that Dr. McSherry and her colleagues argued that the presence of chaplains was more necessary in the DRG era because we (1) helped the hospital reduce the length of stay, (2) cut down the calls for nursing service, and (3) reduced the use of medication. A lot of us, including me, made a beeline to the administration's doorstep with proof of our value. From that moment until today, I am surprised that he did not accept this new evidence with the degree of passion and excitement that I felt. I soon learned his lack of excitement was a portent of things to come. How could this wonderful news be so summarily dismissed?

There have been many studies since, though none have held the degree of excitement and anticipation of final acceptance into the world of medical reimbursement possibilities which that first foray held. One of the most recent was Larry VandeCreek's study (1997) on patient satisfaction. Surely, his study would be an avenue into the kingdom, but unfortunately patient satisfaction by itself could not carry the hopes and dreams of the pastoral care movement on its back.

In fact, the more we deal with this issue the more it seems similar to the problems present in our own personal spiritual searches. One needs to be very certain that s/he is asking a question that helps navigate the journey. Wrong questions can lead us down pathways that take a long time from which to recover. It seems to me that people search for salvation in the words, in the Bible, in the preaching, in hearing the message. If I understand correctly the message of the Judeo-Christian heritage, glimpses of the answer will be found in the process, the act of looking, in the search, and not in any final outcome. I wonder if, like Moses, we will see from afar but never quite get to the promised land.

Scientific research has a little of that quality for me. Research offers some answers to be sure. Like most "gods," these answers have a way of letting us down right when we believe we have discovered the "one true god." To be sure, I have found something very important in the search for the scientific answer. My small engagement of the scientific search has been important, if at times frustrating. Much like our own personal spiritual search, it has become painfully clear to me that we must fully embark upon this sometimes exhausting journey whether we want to or not.

Like the spiritual question, we have no choice but to be involved with the joys and perils of the journey. It is a fact of life. We can ignore thoughtful consideration and purposeful action, but we do so at the peril of the profession. I leave you to draw the analogy of the perils pertaining to our personal spiritual journeys. Along the way I am certain we will discover something about ourselves, about our profession, and about our industry. I suspect, however, we will remain outside the kingdom of the medical world.

So what am I saying? Should we attempt to enter that medical kingdom? Does it mean selling our soul? I believe, and I don't think this is hedging the question that both Chaplain Yes and Chaplain No are right. Chaplain No is right, "Pastoral Care is an art and not a science." However, I do not agree that "such an attempt to sell chaplaincy cannot be accomplished without selling out the every essence of ministry." I do not believe measuring outcomes is selling our soul. At the same time, our reason for being exists outside the healthcare industry and the medical establishment although we function within it. Let there be no mistake—we function in a medical world with a medical model whether we like it or not. What happens inside the doors of a hospital is measured in this modern era by outcomes and financial implications.

One does not need to be very old to know there has been a dramatic shift in healthcare since the institution of DRGs in the early 80s. Since then, health care professionals have been forced to justify their value on the basis of clinical outcomes. I remember the consternation of the physicians suddenly having their medical decisions dictated by protocols rather than the art of medical care. They resisted and still resist practicing medicine by protocol. They do not like being forced into a medical decision by insurance companies who honor a series of scientific outcomes more than the physician's individual judgment.

The demand to follow accepted proven procedures irreversibly changed the nature of medical care, its ethics, its financing, and the physician-patient relationship. Physicians could no longer merely follow a hunch when symptoms did not justify the expenditure of money on tests to follow that hunch. No longer would the hunch be sufficient reason to reimburse the physician or hospital.

The machinations as well as ramifications of this switch to outcomes-based decision-making are enormous. One area it affected most significantly was medical ethics. Discussion of the impact on medical ethics goes beyond the scope of our present task. Suffice it to say that when one makes a decision based on the good of the many versus the good of the individual, the decision and use of resources is often very different. I think it is not too simplistic to say that our medical establishment is groaning under that broad ethical dilemma.

So, regardless of our hopes and dreams, our wishes and preferences, we, like other medical professionals also need to justify the nature and outcome of our work. The manner and nature of that search, of that process is a critical part of this discussion. For me, however, whether that search for outcomes measurements should happen has been resolved.

In preparation for this article, I had some fascinating discussions with the Chief Medical Officer here at this hospital. Dr. Tom Danzi recommended we (the pastoral care profession) follow the lead of the medical profession. He suggests we might have a major high-level conference to establish realistic outcomes for our profession. Once we have agreed upon measurable outcomes, we might then suggest that pastoral care researchers across the nation document and measure these outcomes collaboratively. His prescription for us contains great merit. I believe too many divergent pathways mark the pastoral research landscape. It is important that researchers identify and focus on consensus-based outcomes.

If I use the personal spiritual search analogy referred to above, we are journeying down pathways that carry us far afield from our goal, rather than pathways that justify our services. We are asking questions that are not pertinent to the task. Indeed, it is not clear to me that our profession of pastoral caregiving has focused on the most difficult task as of yet.

A new day has dawned! As physicians needed to prove the outcomes of their ministrations for patients with a variety of illnesses, the use of pathways or protocols became a standard of practice. That standard was tied to physician reimbursement in the managed care model. The treatment pathway mandated, by scientific evidence the treatment by which the patient has the best chance to get better. The DRG revolution in its kindness allowed for increased payment because of severity of illness. These protocols leading to the diagnosis and treatment were determined by large, multi-centered studies across the country. We in the pastoral care profession must have a similar massive undertaking–to prove the value of what we do for patients by more than antidotal material. Factual data is reality in healthcare today.

Neither Dr. Danzi, nor I, underestimates the enormity of the challenge to quantify the value of our services, those that have been thought to be essentially unquantifiable. That is the challenge to pastoral caregivers and our research colleagues. Clearly, we do not have the enormous resources of the medical establishment. But that must not deter us from focusing our questions and our necessary research. The central question facing our profession is "Are there true, definable outcomes that can be validated by data when our primary task is dealing with matters of the heart and soul?" I do not pretend to know the answer, but I believe with heartfelt passion that we must embark upon a unified search.

I am not knowledgeable enough in the limits and scope of research methodology to know exactly how to do it. However, I think there have been many attempts by serious experts in the field of statistical analysis. I believe we need to follow up the studies of researchers such as McSherry, Vandecreek, Larsen, Pargament, Koenig as well as others with one or two major well-developed nationally coordinated multi-centered studies.

At this hospital Dr. Saurabh Chokshi, a Hindu cardiologist, believes his studies have demonstrated that patients who received spiritual counseling have done much better after by-pass surgery. The group that received counseling had fewer incidents of irregular heart rhythms and needed less pain medication–McSherry's study revisited 15 years later.

The Business News of Tampa Bay (2001, p. 4) recently quoted Dr. Chokshi as saying, "If providing spiritual care means people recover quicker and leave the hospital sooner, it has the potential of saving hundreds of thousands of dollars."

We have a number of brilliant scientists who believe they have shown beyond doubt how spiritual care has meant savings in pain and expense, as well as increased patient satisfaction and fewer lawsuits.

We must, as a profession, undertake research as physicians did, especially after the initiation of the DRG era. They researched their treatment protocols and determined their effectiveness. They proved to the medical community and to the public which treatment decisions were most efficacious.

I believe we can prove that the presence of a chaplain is not only well received by the patient and family, but also cost efficient, and worthy of significant financial support. The only way that will happen, however, is through a nationwide, multi-centered research protocol, accepted by the most skeptical scientists as solid in its procedures and therefore, its outcomes. To be sure, funding such a major study will be expensive and, perhaps resisted by some. However, the blending of sensitive spiritual care, individualized to maximize each person's coping skills, with state of the art medicine can, I believe, be a most significant breakthrough of this 21st century.

We need to gain a clear focus of the journey, indeed the spiritual journey of our profession in hospitals. Those of us in chaplaincy know that we are critically important to many people. Indeed, all of us have had experiences where we knew our relationship was as important, if not more important to the overall health of the patient and family than the medical care they received. And don't forget the benefit to the staff of this kind of sensitive pastoral presence. Clearly these are not isolated events. I believe we can prove that through consistent applied multi-centered research conducted simultaneously across the country. May our pathways remain straight!

REFERENCES

The Business Journal. (December 14-29, 2001), page 4.

McSherry, E., Kratz, D., & Nelson, Wm. (1986). Pastoral Care Departments: More necessary in the DRG era? *HCMR 11*(1), 47-59.

VandeCreek, L. (1997). *Ministry of Hospital Chaplains: Patient Satisfaction.* New York: The Haworth Press, Inc.

To Be, Or Not To Be More Scientific?
That Is the Question:
Yes, Absolutely, But . . .

Paul Steven Bay, DMin, BCC

SUMMARY. I use a systems theory approach to address the question of whether or not to become more scientific in our professions of pastoral education and chaplaincy. While acknowledging and discussing the many tensions and issues raised by this important question, I provide a rationale for why we must become more scientific. I reflect on the costs of both becoming more scientific and not becoming more scientific in our professions. *[Article copies available for a fee from The Haworth Document Delivery Service: 1-800-HAWORTH. E-mail address: <docdelivery@haworthpress.com> Website: <http://www.HaworthPress.com> © 2002 by The Haworth Press, Inc. All rights reserved.]*

KEYWORDS. Chaplaincy, pastoral care, clinical pastoral education, scientific research, systems theory

This Christmas holiday season I had a new experience. When I placed our angels in the yard, one set of lights on one angel wouldn't work. After some preliminary tests to make sure I had electricity to the

---

Paul Steven Bay is Cardiovascular Services Chaplain, Chaplaincy and Pastoral Education, Clarian/Methodist Hospital, I-65 at 21st Street, P.O. Box 1367, Indianapolis, IN 46206-1367 (E-mail: pbay@clarian.com).

[Haworth co-indexing entry note]: "To Be, Or Not To Be More Scientific? That Is the Question: Yes, Absolutely, But . . ." Bay, Paul Steven. Co-published simultaneously in *Journal of Health Care Chaplaincy* (The Haworth Pastoral Press, an imprint of The Haworth Press, Inc.) Vol. 12, No. 1/2, 2002, pp. 19-27; and: *Professional Chaplaincy and Clinical Pastoral Education Should Become More Scientific: Yes and No* (ed: Larry VandeCreek) The Haworth Pastoral Press, an imprint of The Haworth Press, Inc., 2003, pp. 19-27. Single or multiple copies of this article are available for a fee from The Haworth Document Delivery Service [1-800-HAWORTH, 9:00 a.m. - 5:00 p.m. (EST). E-mail address: docdelivery@haworthpress.com].

10.1300/J080v12n01_03

sockets I went to a nearby store and bought 100 replacement six-volt bulbs. To replace a bulb I stripped the bulb from the old base, ran the two wires on the new bulb through their respective holes and put the new bulb in the socket. I did this with a hundred bulbs and the lights still did not come on. At that point I tried one of these new bulbs in a socket where a bulb was burning. To my surprise the new bulb did not light up. It was then that I decided maybe I had the wrong size bulbs. I went to another store and found replacement bulbs that said 2 1/2-volts. The package of 2 1/2-volt bulbs clearly said it was for 100-strand bulbs and I discovered my 6-volt package said it was for 35-count strands. I thought of the chapter title "Sharpen the Saw" in *The Seven Habits of Highly Effective People* (Stephen Covey, 1989). I had been sawing without sharpening the saw and I had wasted a lot of energy.

This metaphor comes to mind as I think about the place of research in the field of chaplaincy. Rather than jump right in, the question deserves pondering. My sharpening the saw is the pondering of this question by raising many more questions. In this paper I will use the terms "research" and "becoming more scientific" interchangeably. They mean an intentional examination of disciplined or methodical ways of providing pastoral education or pastoral care.

My training in systems theory calls for me to step back and look at research in chaplaincy and Clinical Pastoral Education (CPE) from the largest perspective I can. I recall the wisdom of Rabbi Edwin Friedman. His teaching about anxiety within systems and our tendency to be reactive to lessen the anxiety is instructive. I don't want to say "Yes" or "No" to CPE and chaplaincy becoming more scientific merely as a reaction to health care reform or because I feel pressure to help my hospital be listed in *U.S. News and World Reports' 100 Best Hospitals*. The decision to be more scientific or to not be more scientific, in my practice as a chaplain, is too important to be an anxiety-driven decision.

I once wrote an article integrating a couple of ideas from Robert Bly and Craig Dykstra. The writing of both men came to mind around the issue of becoming more scientific in chaplaincy and CPE. Dykstra's (1996) ideas around "A Long Obedience in the Same Direction" will be addressed later. Robert Bly's thinking that spoke to me came from a chapter titled "The Long Bag We Drag Behind Us" in *A Little Book on the Human Shadow* (1988). He talks about the Bly boys having bags a mile long by the time they were twelve. What are some of the thoughts in the long bag I, as a chaplain, drag behind me? I offer six for our reflection, although like the Bly boys there are many more in my bag.

First, I often experience chaplains and pastoral educators believing that what they do cannot be measured. Furthermore, I sometimes find myself glad no one has said I must measure my ministry. This gives me a lot of freedom to define my ministry myself. I have often thought of the amount of time a nurse spends giving bedside care and been thankful I can teach, read some or make phone calls. I do not have to constantly be with patients. My understanding of healing further complicates measuring ministry. I see healing as being done from the inside out. I see myself as supporting and facilitating healing. How can these be measured?

A second item in the long bag is the state of health care as I experience it. I define it in part as a dysfunctional system. I have both been taught and have learned by experience that the only way to stay healthy in a dysfunctional system is to define myself and stay in touch with the system. To define myself means for me to decide whether or not research is a part of my calling and my responsibility as a chaplain or pastoral educator. I also know that I do nothing from pure motives. One way to see this clearly is to view the basis of why I do research on a continuum. Picture satisfying administration on one end of the continuum; my commitment to be a responsible professional would be on the other end. It makes a world of difference where my motivation comes from on that continuum. Few of us would be totally on one end or the other.

The second part of the way to stay healthy is to "stay in touch with the system." Staying in touch with the system invites the question, "Is being more scientific a necessity to stay in touch with my health care peers such as physicians, nurses and therapists?" A second question comes to mind, "How can I stay in touch if I can't speak the language of the other health care team?"

Another reality of the health care system today is expressed by Gatchil and Maddrey (1998). "The cost-effectiveness of a particular therapeutic modality is becoming increasingly important in today's environment of managed care" (p. 36-42). How good am I at showing I'm cost effective? A third item is the long bag is awareness that my profession is born out of Anton Boisen and other leaders of the CPE movement looking at ministry to the sick differently than their colleagues. Indeed Boisen's process was more scientific than his peers in ministry. Coupled with this is the knowledge that as a chaplain I am part of a larger system (health care) that is in constant change. Peter Steinke's (1996) words bear heavy on my mind: "All living systems are endangered when they lack flexibility" (p. 69). What might it cost my patients, the health care system and me if I choose to be inflexible?

A fourth item in the long bag is the question of my view of my ministry. Do I view myself in the prophetic role of ministering to the health of the health care system itself? To what extent can I see health care as the identified patient to whom I minister? As a trained therapist, as well as chaplain, I am aware that there is an objectivity of being on the edge of a system rather than in the throes of the dynamic processes occurring within the system. This position gives me better leverage to be an agent of change. Is it possible that I could facilitate greater health in the health care system by not being caught up in measuring what I do from a scientific stance? Would this position of not using the same methodology as my health care peers be a plus?

A fifth item in the long bag is the historical context of health care and chaplaincy. Some chaplains have lost their jobs because their value to the health care system was not clearly enough defined, understood, or communicated. On the other hand there is the experience of two groups: physicians and social workers. They have defined themselves more specifically as a result of health care reform. Unfortunately, higher role definition has reduced job satisfaction and fulfillment considerably for both groups. Is losing my job in health care a real possibility? Is losing my job satisfaction and fulfillment a real likelihood?

A final item in my long bag is growth. Growth was a value emphasized in clinical pastoral education (CPE). It has remained a value for me as a chaplain. Yet, is my own desire for growth sufficient for me to give my best pastoral care? Does my energy for providing excellent pastoral care or pastoral education wax and wane? Do I need the discipline of research and the learning that comes from the results research provides? Do I need to become more scientific in my approach in order to do "best practices"?

Research utilizing a more scientific approach to religion and spirituality in health care is already being done. It is significant that physicians, psychologists and professionals other than chaplains are taking leadership roles in this research. How do I feel about this? Does my role call for me to be leader in this work and its publication?

Remember Don Quixote? Do I suffer from a quixotic complex? Do I feel chaplains are the only health care professionals left who can and do go into patients' rooms and listen as they express their feelings, needs, hopes, and grief? Am I the only human element of health care left? Is my profession the last holdout? Remember the Alamo! If I start being more scientific and doing research then am I on a slippery slope? Will my devotion to "the living human document" be swallowed up?

Steinke (1996) quotes Sir William Osler who said, "It is more important to know what sort of patient has the disease than what sort of disease the patient has" (p. 23). Having read recently that the Ebola virus has again broken out in Gabon Africa reminds me that linear thinking like Osler's statement doesn't provide enough truth. It also reminds me that I, even as a chaplain, can be guilty of linear thinking, just as I have sometimes thought of scientists. I seriously doubt that knowing who the person is affects the survival rate in Ebola that causes death in 50%-90% of all cases. On the other hand knowing the patient when I was nine years old and diagnosed with an ulcer probably would have helped. I needed glasses and didn't know it, and I was having a terrible time with grades in school. Much of the time healing calls for knowing both the patient and the disease but this is not always true.

Can chaplaincy and pastoral education be an art that is both scientific and compassionate? My limited experience doing research, and extensive experience as a clinician says chaplaincy can be both. My observation of pastoral educators and co-leading groups with them says pastoral education can be both. Professionals in both fields can utilize scientific method and still address an individual's needs with deep caring. This highlights one perspective problem into which I sometimes fall; polarizing scientific method and compassion. These are not opposites!

Some events push me to be truthful with myself regarding my commitment to my profession. I recall a sense of uncomfortable surprise when I discovered that the authors Paul Pruyser and Michael Cavanagh were psychologists, people in a profession other than ministry that wrote outstanding works on ministry. (I am aware that there are many outstanding books by chaplains defining our ministry.) I have similar feelings when I see much of the literature on the effects of religion or spirituality being written by physicians. CPE supervisors Art Lucas and his colleagues (2001) have challenged me to think about my intention in giving pastoral care with their work with *The Discipline*. I wonder why health care providers had to start talking about "best practices" before I began to examine more clearly my "best practices"? I think it only honest to admit many other professional chaplains and I have not worked very hard at integrating scientific methodology into the practice of chaplaincy to improve our ministry.

I have not been diligent in learning more about scientific inquiry and found it helpful to consult various dictionaries for the definition of science. In general, it is: (1) The observation, identification, description, experimental investigation, and theoretical explanation of phenomena. (2) Methodological activity, discipline or study. (3) An activity regarded as requiring study and method. (4) Knowledge gained through experience. I believe CPE-trained chaplains have been using scientific methods for a long time. All chaplains I know are using observation, identifying things like needs, hopes, resources, using description of faith experiences and seeking to gain knowledge through their experiences. However, I have challenged myself to do research because I am weak in being methodical. A limited understanding of research has paralleled my limited understanding of science. I now know there are a number of research methods besides quantitative approaches. A helpful start in understanding research is *Research in Pastoral Care and Counseling: Quantitative and Qualitative Approaches* (VandeCreek, Bender & Jordon, 1994).

For much of my career as a chaplain I was not concerned with our profession becoming more scientific. Furthermore, there was no pressure to become more methodical or disciplined in my chaplaincy. In my CPE experience, writing verbatims and case studies was using scientific methods but was never called scientific. I was required to do a research project but was taught very little about research methodology.

There is a lot more in the long bag, but the question "Should clinical pastoral education and chaplaincy become more scientific?" begs an answer. My answer is "Yes, absolutely, but." I must be more scientific in my approach, but I must act from a proactive stance. I do research because it fits my value that chaplaincy and CPE are disciplined arts. I believe I owe it to my patients and myself because it is essential for "best practices." I am unaware of a better way to be disciplined or improve my art than scientific inquiry.

However, this decision is made with many unanswered questions. Can there be a healthy integration of the business model, medical model, social science and theological models in delivery of health care? Are all the models with which we have experimented to date too limiting? Does measuring what we do have potential to be a problem in that we become too numbers conscious and detail oriented? Does not measuring what we do leave us open to other health care workers defining us primarily through their own projections? Does not measuring what we do leave us in the dark as to what we really are doing and how well we do it?

What if our research doesn't prove we make a difference in length of stay, use of pain medication, recovery, or other aspects of healing? If we set a protocol or standard that a patient is at a particular point on the third day post-operatively are we manipulating the patient to meet our need? Could we be putting God in a box if we decide what spiritual health looks like on the third day post-operatively? Does research improve knowledge or practice, neither or both?

A more fundamental question concerns whether we have tried to create a healing environment. If the purpose of a hospital were to be a healing community what would be the characteristics and skills of the people selected? Are there pieces of human experience we don't know how to measure through research? Is there a danger of deifying research and making it a larger part of the picture than it should be? Do we have to be able to read and understand scientific articles to be informed health care team members?

Where does our power come from? Does each person have a unique individual spirit? If so, can one carry out research and still capture some of that individual spirit? How important is relationship in the context of healing? If responsible chaplaincy calls for the integration of an art and scientific method, are both art and science inexact and always changing? How well have we demonstrated that we make a difference? If healing is the body's potential to repair and regenerate itself, do we know how to research our assisting this process? What interventions most promote healing? Is asking questions a form of research?

Earlier in this article I referred to the influence of Craig Dykstra (1996), Vice President for Religion with the Lilly Endowment who wrote a piece called "A Long Obedience in the Same Direction." His point is that the essential thing in life is to have a guiding star so we can stay on track, or find our way again, when we get off track. It seems to me this expression embodies the best response to what chaplaincy and CPE should be. Let's look at some of the issues I have raised with the question in mind of what a long obedience in the right direction would be.

1. Can what we do be measured? To a large extent we could measure the outcomes and results of many of our pastoral interventions. We can probably measure some of the healing that occurs from the inside out. For example, we can measure whether or not a pastoral intervention increases hope which does help the healing process. I think we can measure our assistance in the grief process and develop better tools to measure relationship dynamics such as reconciliation that we can facilitate.

2. We can reflect on our own motivation and commitment to improving our profession through clearer data. Is it not part of the value "to love my neighbor" which compels me to know, practice, and share more scientific data about how spiritual care and pastoral education makes a difference? How will our health care peers

such as doctors, nurses, respiratory therapists and others learn that we help with the healing process unless we share publications and do research?

3. Do we have both an obligation and opportunity to embrace the challenge of change in healthcare, by being open to new forms of ministry as our CPE founding fathers were?

4. We have specialized training in relational dynamics and several chaplains and pastoral educators are trained in system dynamics. Health care has become an imbalanced system. The business model has taken dominance. We could take the lead in modeling balancing research and care. We could be the change agents the health care system needs.

5. We need to answer the questions of what we do and how cost effective we are. We know best who we are and what we do. Passively resisting the scientific process as a part of what we do, leaves us vulnerable to be defined by others such as managed care. Furthermore, if we do not provide some cost effectiveness we probably should not be labeled health care professionals. If you are as convinced as I am that we do save our hospitals dollars then the question really becomes, "Are we diligent enough to demonstrate our financial effect?"

6. Does research improve knowledge or practice, neither or both? I think that even a cursory look at the practice of medicine answers this question. Knowledge obtained primarily through research has added unbelievably to medicine. Having just experienced laparascopic hernia surgery, I find the practice of medicine to have improved too. This is one of thousands of practices made less painful and less burdensome in the healing process.

7. Final questions I offer relate to the creation story. Do you believe the world was created in six days or do you espouse the scientific evidence that it was a more lengthy process? If like me you espouse that scientific process has offered a good deal of truth about the creation process, has that lessened your belief that God is indeed our world's creator? My point is that scientific teaching is not the enemy or opposite of the Biblical account and our faith in God as creator. I can comfortably hold the scientific belief of creation and faith in God as creator. Scientific method is not the opposite of, or enemy of chaplaincy or CPE. It offers tools and perspective that can enhance and work with our compassionate caring.

I realize it is a major characteristic of our linear thinking that we want answers. The question of should chaplaincy and clinical pastoral education be more scientific in response to health care raises more questions than it answers. However, the pastoral care literature of the last few years has made real strides in addressing many of these questions. The work describing "The Discipline" (VandeCreek & Lucas, 2001) is a good example of a long obedience in the same direction. My article has focused on clinical questions faced by chaplains and pastoral educators. It has offered a very limited view of the social context of tensions between science and professions such as ours. A more complete discussion of these tensions can be found in the works of Ken Wilber (2000).

We live in a systemic world. As Peter Steinke (1996) puts it so well, "Systems thinking is basically a way of thinking about life as all of a piece" (p. 3). So my answer to this question is "Yes, absolutely, but." The "but" will not go away because this question is complex and multi-faceted. The question is so important that it must be revisited often. The reason behind our answer is as important as the answer. The questions raised can be a doorway to better clarify our answers. Most importantly, the outcome will be the potential to practice our professions of chaplaincy and pastoral educators to the best of our ability.

REFERENCES

Bly, R. (1988). *A Little Book on the Human Shadow*. New York: HarperCollins Publishers, p. 17.

Covey, S. (1989). *The Seven Habits of Highly Effective People: Restoring the Character Ethic*. New York: Simon & Schuster, p. 287.

Dykstra, Craig. (Spring 1996). A long obedience in the same direction. *Initiatives in Religion,* 5 (#2) 1-2.

Gatchel, R. & Maddrey, A. (Sept. 1998). Clinical outcome research in complementary and alternative medicine: An overview of experimental design and analysis. *Alternative Therapies*, 4 (5), 36-42.

Steinke, Peter L. (1996). *Healthy Congregations: A Systems Approach*. New York: The Alban Institute.

Vandecreek, Larry, Hilary Bender and Merle Jordon. (1994). *Research in Pastoral Care and Counseling: Quantitative and Qualitative Approaches*. Journal of Pastoral Care Publications, Inc.

VandeCreek, Larry and Arthur Lucas, editors. (2001). The discipline for pastoral care giving: Foundations for outcome oriented chaplaincy. *Journal of Health Care Chaplaincy*. New York: The Haworth Pastoral Press, 10 (#2).

Wilber, Ken. (2000). *A Brief History of Everything*. Boston, MA: Shambhala Publications, Inc.

Chaplains and Science

W. Noel Brown, STM, BCC

SUMMARY. The decision between science and religion is eroding. The changing relationship is associated with the discovery of similarities between science and religion. Chaplains must become more comfortable with science and let it inform our ministry. *[Article copies available for a fee from The Haworth Document Delivery Service: 1-800-HAWORTH. E-mail address: <docdelivery@haworthpress.com> Website: <http://www.HaworthPress.com> © 2002 by The Haworth Press, Inc. All rights reserved.]*

KEYWORDS. Chaplaincy, pastoral care, science, clinical pastoral education

Science is the highest form of adoration.[1]

So Teilhard de Chardin, Jesuit priest and scientist

W. Noel Brown is Editor, The Orere Source, P.O. Box 362, Harbert MI 49115 and Chaplain Supervisor, Northwestern Memorial Hospital, Chicago, IL 60611 (E-mail: oreresource@rocketmail.com).

[Haworth co-indexing entry note]: "Chaplains and Science." Brown, W. Noel. Co-published simultaneously in *Journal of Health Care Chaplaincy* (The Haworth Pastoral Press, an imprint of The Haworth Press, Inc.) Vol. 12, No. 1/2, 2002, pp. 29-41; and: *Professional Chaplaincy and Clinical Pastoral Education Should Become More Scientific: Yes and No* (ed: Larry VandeCreek) The Haworth Pastoral Press, an imprint of The Haworth Press, Inc., 2003, pp. 29-41. Single or multiple copies of this article are available for a fee from The Haworth Document Delivery Service [1-800-HAWORTH, 9:00 a.m. - 5:00 p.m. (EST). E-mail address: docdelivery@haworthpress.com].

10.1300/J080v12n01_04

AN INTRODUCTION BY WAY OF A CONFESSION

I begin with a confession. I am a board certified chaplain and an Association for Clinical Pastoral Education (ACPE) supervisor. However, I am also a scientist. My first degree was in pure and applied chemistry and the training for that degree provided me with experiences that have subsequently influenced my work both as a chaplain and as a supervisor. That training taught me certain values that affect my reflections on my interactions with people and the world. I disclose this "conflict of interest" to alert you to the fact that I have a bias. I have been working scientifically as a minister, chaplain and supervisor for over thirty-five years.

THE SEPARATION OF SCIENCE AND RELIGION

In the 1960s when I was a science undergraduate, there was considerable debate about the relationship between science and religion. It was an era in which science was enjoying unparalleled support and making great claims for what it would contribute to the future of humankind. The transistor had been invented. The potential of nuclear reactions for good (and ill) was being recognized. The fuel cell had been invented though hardly perfected. "The pill" had been formulated. "Better living through chemistry" and "What won't they think of next" were the slogans of an era when people in the Western world were coming to believe that it was science that had all the answers to the problems of the world. It might take a little time, but science was going to reign supreme. On the other hand, religion was on the defensive as people started to believe that science could eventually overcome mystery. "God is dead" claimed a cover of *Time* Magazine.[2]

Then an interesting development began to unfold. Following the boundless optimism of the 1960s, it took little more than a generation to discover that science did not have all the answers, and in fact, many discoveries often brought with them significant problems that no amount of science could ever answer. As the western world's infatuation with the potential of science began to fade in the 70s and 80s, a strange twist began to occur in the relationship between science and religion. It began to be suggested that, in fact, science is itself a religious enterprise, both science and religion sharing many characteristics in common. When the structure of scientific investigation began to be examined, it was seen that science is grounded implicitly in a fundamental faith stance–a faith in truth and value. In the steps of the scientific method, science is seen to move with a faithful confidence towards greater and clearer understanding. Science, or more accurately, "the scientific method" observes reality as best it can, and then by leaps of the imagination that are sometimes heavily reasoned, sometimes intuitive, it creates images, symbols, theories to express its experiences. We call them experiments, which are accompanied by the process of linking up what is already known, describing what now has been newly discovered, and sometimes offering hints about the future.

Most people even today have not realized that religion and science have much in common. Many, including chaplains are influenced by the popular beliefs about science that have long obscured both the religious and the imaginative aspects of science. In 1883 Ernst Mach published his influential book *Die Mechanik in ihrer Entwicklung* (*The Development of Mechanics*) in which he stated what many persons thought at that time and what many still believe today: that science is a passionless observation of brute facts, a detached observation of the activities of the world and people.[3] Mach maintained that science should only be coldly objective and rational, devoid of feeling or bias. In fact this was really his Teutonic bias. Much of science and many scientific discoveries have been the result of leaps of the imagination and dreams–both by day and night. Such discoveries are then received and discussed within communities of faith, which we know as "schools of psychology," "branches of physics," "academies of physicians."

While Mach was encouraging the public and his scientific colleagues to believe that the scientific enterprise involves objective observations of the world, Friedrich Schleiermarcher (1768-1834) was taking religion in the opposite direction. He asserted that religious faith, specifically the Christian faith, is not to be found in objective observations of the world of persons, nor could it even be found in rational thinking about beliefs and morality. He argued that true religion is located in inner experience, and vision.

So as the western world entered the 20th century, the division between science and religion was clear. Science was characterized by impersonal objectivity. Religion was related to inner experience. This dichotomy was reinforced by some of the great minds of the first half of the 20th century. The great philosopher, essayist and peace advocate Bertrand Russell (1872-1970) believed that scientific statements are always based on external evidence, and that religion is based on inner emotions and moral feelings. Wittgenstein, his pupil concluded that religion and science are two separate and distinct kinds of language enterprises, each with its own logic, different and separate from each other. So a split that had begun around 1600 had led to a situation by the early 1960s where orthodox science and orthodox religion deeply distrusted, and often despised each other.

THE PLACE OF IMAGINATION IN SCIENCE

Since the late middle of the 20th century, the division between science and religion has been seriously eroding. The narrow reductionistic view of science characterized by Mach, Russell and Wittgenstein is now seen as outmoded, even though it lingers in the modern mind. Post-Heisenberg, we are more circumspect in the way we understand "reality." There is an acceptance of the fact that central to our explanations of reality are models or paradigms which are used for both theory and practice. It has also been realized that these models are the products of the human imagination. What scientists create are "imaginative constructs invented to account for observed phenomena."[4] The imagination of the scientist has a very important creative function, not just in imagining, but also in creativity. Paul Ricouer points out that the birth of metaphors (i.e., models) arise from creative collisions of the imaginative acts of people exploring their worlds, who bring and hold together contradictory meanings, and that when these meanings come together ("collide") they in turn create new meanings. Ricoeur puts it this way: "are we not ready to recognize in the power of imagination, no longer the faculty of deriving 'images' from our sensory experience, but the capacity for letting new worlds shape our understanding of ourselves."[5]

The history of the social and hard sciences is replete with examples of scientists who were imaginatively involved with their research that led to so-called "breakthroughs" in their work. Albert Einstein had an almost mystical involvement with his work. Mendeleyev finally understood the ordering of the periodic table in a dream. Galileo imagined the nature of motion in a way completely at odds with everyone else of his day, imagining a model that became the basis for Newton's laws of thermodynamics. Milton Erickson's insight that behavioral change could be fostered by encouraging patient restraint had its origins when as a 7-year old he pulled on the tail of a cow that was refusing to enter his father's barn. Now where did that idea come from? Great scientists have been and are truly creative. They work in tune with their own inner reality. They identify with what they are trying to understand. Their attitudes, intuitions, feelings and aesthetic sensitivities are as much involved in their science as counting and fact gathering. Their science involves their whole person, rather than just a capacity for dispassionate objectification.

There is a secret concerning the scientific community that is little known by outsiders. It involves a division within that community. In one group are those who are followers of Francis Bacon (1561-1626), who did his science in order to "control nature." They are the command and control crowd. In the second group are the followers of Adam Smith (1723-1790), an economist/philosopher who wrote about the study of the world in what was to be a major work and which was only published after his death (*Essays on Philosophical Subjects,* published 1795). About his own understanding of the scientific method he wrote: "Wonder, therefore, and not any expectation of advantage from its discoveries, is the first principle which *promp*ts mankind to the study of Philosophy, of that science which pretends to lay open the concealed connections that unite the various appearance of nature; and they pursue this study for its own sake, as an original pleasure or good in itself, without regarding its tendency to procure them the means of many other pleasures."[6] He leads the contemplate and confess crowd. Teilhard de Chardin would be a member of this second group. "Perhaps . . . We shall end by perceiving that the great object unconsciously pursued by science is nothing else than the discovery of God."[7] So would my old mathematics professor. In one of our lectures, he completed a long mathematical equation. It covered several blackboards and took about 30 minutes to deduce and write. He then stood back and talked not about the mathematics he had just derived, but about the "beauty" of what he had just demonstrated. In private he would speak of the world of mathematics in explicitly religious terms.

SIMILARITIES IN THE PRACTICES
OF SCIENCE AND RELIGION

So far we have suggested that the world of science is not a world of dispassion and rationality as is commonly thought. In fact, the more closely one looks at the behavior of a creative scientist the more that person looks like a religious believer. I contend that this is not surprising in that both science and religion are fundamentally remarkably parallel enterprises.

Both religion and science deal with mystery–the unknown and the unfamiliar. Both communities have a commitment to seeking the truth as well as a faith that truth can be found. Scientists have faith in regularity and patterns of the universe. They have faith that knowledge is possible. They have faith that new truth will reveal itself if they prepare themselves and their experiments carefully. Faith is a foundation of science, just as it is of religion and chaplaincy. Scientists act like believers. The dedicated scientist has a positive attitude toward reality, all of that parallels the Judaeo-Christian stance towards the world of creation– "the earth is the Lord's and the fullness thereof." Science and religion both believe that there is a truth to be sought and to be found, a truth whose attainment comes through the pursuit of well-motivated belief.

The scientist carries within him/herself a sense of the importance and the appropriateness of the scientific pursuit of knowledge. It is their calling, just as the religious person is committed to doing what they believe they have been called to do. Both groups, out of a sense of faith about who they are, what they are doing, and what they are seeking, move forward toward new discoveries, believing there is something to be found at the end, that they do not live and work within a vacuum, but within a total order or world-view which can only be labeled as worthwhile. To paraphrase Dag Hammerskjold who might have said about the faith of both groups: "Behind all of their desire and application is an Infinite Yes."

The best in both have an attitude of openness, to imaginatively exploring new ideas. This is why Islamic science withered and died when their religious fundamentalists in the 11th century limited the quest for new knowledge, not allowing open thought.[8]

Last, but most important, individuals in both groups are part of a larger community of faith. The religious communities and the scientific communities exhibit notably parallel behaviors concerning the place of the individual and their relationship to the larger group. Both gather together to share their experiences, engage in ritual practices such as entry rites and memorial rites, each work at clarifying meanings so that they can talk with one another, and they often work to exclude heretics.

The more closely one examines the behavior of a good scientist, the more they may look like a religious believer.

SOME NEW SCIENTIFIC METHODS

Ken Wilber, the transpersonal philosopher, has made a strong case that new understandings of the world do not have to come via the methods of traditional science. He argues that there are three types of science and that each type is appropriate for one of the three main domains that together comprise reality as we know it today. First there is the domain that we know by means of our senses. It is the domain which traditional science has claimed as its own and exploited with such great success. The second domain is the one we can only access with our "inner eye." Social (or mental) science–Europeans call it Geisfeswissenschaft–does not observe objects using the senses, but explores the data–in this case, meanings–which can be found in documents, stories, books, myths, reports. The meaning of a text is not found by the physical eye, only with the "eye of reason." The third domain is the Self, the principle in us that sees and thinks. It cannot be seen and is not a thought, and even it can be studied experimentally in meditation. Meditation itself can be understood as a scientific method because it follows the three strands of Kuhn in his description of the processes which together comprise the scientific method: (1) Injunction/Instruction. (2) Illumination/Observation. (3) Confirmation. "It is a mistake to fall into the old and now discarded belief that science (meaning the objective, reductionist approach to exploring the world) is the only road to understanding, the royal route to reality, and the only true source of dependable knowledge. It is now accepted that there are a number of different doors to gaining data about different aspects of our world."[9]

Over the last 20 years, new ways of trying to understand "reality" have been created especially for the second domain. Some of them not only look different from the style of the "uninvolved observer" approach, they also intuitively feel welcoming for chaplains. A good example is the method devised by Glauser and Strauss.[10] Their method includes the gathering of stories that are then examined in various disciplined ways in order to be able to gain new insights and to identify new models of understanding. Their work has been found to be of value by nurses, social workers, and chaplains who are working to understand what happens both within and between persons.

Another method is known as participatory research. This style of research starts with the active participation together of researcher (the object) and the person(s) being researched (the objects). It began in international development work, but has been found to be valuable in health care settings. Collaboration, education and action are the key elements of this form of research. It is based on a mutually respectful partnership between researchers and communities–a far cry from the dispassionate non-involvement of traditional science.[11]

Having noted all these, we should add that there is also still knowledge to be gained from traditional scientific work, as Iler and his colleagues demonstrated in their recent study published in *Chaplaincy Today*.[12] When examined, their method too can be seen to follow the steps of Kuhn (op. cit.11) and shows how traditional science still holds much of value for the development of more effective ministry·

SCIENCE IS AN ART, NOT A SCIENCE

Whether the field of endeavor is in the world of our senses, the world of mental experiences or the world of religious or spiritual experiences, the fruits in each field are the result of imaginative attempts to interpret reality. All are built on lesser interpretations, and they are made on the basis of a foundational faith, as we have described above. What makes traditional science stand apart from, say, religion and spirituality is that is has chosen to claim that it is only certain methods of data-acquisition which are reliable, namely, its own. It also has procedures that allow behavior to be repeated, as if repetition was an indication that repetition provides a firmer grasp on truth or reality. Direct experience and repeated behavior in other fields, for example, discoveries in meditation or the inner feelings of persons have been rejected as inadequate experiential evidence for "scientific purposes." But if we accept that the basic structure of the scientific method as it was first suggested by Kuhn,[13] we can see these same processes are possible in all three domains of human enquiry: the world we see with our senses; the world we see with our inner eye; and, the world which does the seeing–the Self. In each of these domains, we can do what Kuhn identified only in the domain of the senses. First, we follow an instruction. Second, we perceive a certain state of affairs. Third, we compare our findings to those of others. It is a pattern not dissimilar to the action-reflection model of CPE! To fit the CPE process inside Wilber's understanding of the way valid knowledge is obtained, we start with an injunction: "If you want to know, do this." This is followed by experience of the data from the doing. Finally, there is a checking of the data, the evidence, with the help of others who have completed the first two steps for themselves.[14] It is an action-reflection model.

So, what does it mean for a chaplain to think scientifically? The process of science involves fully attending to some aspect of reality using a process appropriate to what is being considered. Then, based on the interaction (experiment), constructing a model that will be the basis for helping others to understand what we know about that reality, that is, telling a story about it to a group of people who are interested in the same kinds of stories, because they too are involved in the same arena of interest. In order to come to a reality and fully attend to it involves several other prior activities by way of preparation. The researcher talks with others–perhaps by reading those who have had or have an interest in that same part of reality. There will often be conversation (actual or by reading) with others who have anything to say which may assist the encounter, to see if there is anything to be learned from what others have done or found could not be done.

THE RELUCTANCE OF CHAPLAINS TO BE "SCIENTIFIC"

Why have chaplains been so resistant to making connections and building models related to their ministry, especially when they have been so strongly encouraged in their training to deal with the "ordinary," especially the ordinary world of feelings and meanings, to be attentive to and perceptive of both the inner and outer worlds? Training for ministry has been primarily a cognitive exercise. It was for this reason that CPE came in to being, in reaction to the overwhelmingly cognitive and didactic style of the early 20th century seminary, a style that remains largely unchanged today in some US seminaries. Students still come to CPE having received a fixed body of information by means of "banking," or "jug" pedagogy.[15] The educational methods of CPE have rightly remained in apposition to such a cognitive approach. At the same time, CPE has resisted the challenge of conceptualizing issues of expertise and competence in the performance of ministry. Considered, for example, the protracted difficulty within ACPE to define the differences between Level 1 and Level 2 CPE. There are skills and techniques involved in the exercise of ministry. Knowledge is important. Some CPE students routinely recoil when they realize that they are required to actually learn and then impart specific information about, for example, advance directives, not because such material is linked to mortality, but because they have to learn precisely what certain things mean, and be able to explain them very precisely. The practice of pastoral assessment is also not always readily accepted. ("Isn't that being judgmental?" is often a student response.)

A second but related reason may be related to the different inner processes used by persons to process external data. A high percentage of persons who are drawn to ministry, including chaplaincy, have personality "types" such that they do not feel at home in an environment, where external specificity is important. The (frequent) INFPs of the chaplaincy world are quite different from the (frequent) INTJs of the scientific world.

A third reason why some in the church (so I presume some chaplains) have been suspicious about science is their fear that as our knowledge about various aspects of reality increases, we will lose our ability to marvel, to wonder, to be moved by these "understood" aspects of reality. It need not. For me, in fact, exactly the opposite appears to be true. Knowing the mathematics of a rainbow has not decreased my feelings of delight when I see one. I can describe the chemistry of a porcelain glaze on a piece of pottery, but knowing how that effect was achieved does not diminish my enjoyment of the beauty of the pot.

A fourth reason is the lack of training in the field of research during one's preparation for ministry, both in seminaries and in CPE. It is not a requirement for certification in the Association for Professional Chaplains, though some have been proposing that it should be.

CONCLUSION

We have not been afraid of the discoveries made by others, we have welcomed the fruits of their science. Was Kubler-Ross functioning as a scientist when she first wrote about caring for the dying, and described her so-called "stages of dying"? Yes. In some earlier work she had done with schizophrenics, based on her observations, she thought that she saw "stages" in their illnesses. It was that insight that she brought in her looking at the process of dying.[16] The rest is history. Clergy and chaplains have not been reluctant to make use of her "scientific" observations about the "stages" of dying, even though her model is now quite discredited.[17] Nor have we been reluctant to learn from the models created by Carl Rogers (non-directive listening), or Carl Jung (dreams and the unconscious), Harry Stack Sullivan (inter-personal relations), or Paul Pruyser (pastoral diagnoses), all of whom, interestingly, were from outside the field of pastoral care.

We need not be afraid of being disciplined in reflecting on our ministry. This is what we teach our students to do in CPE. We have them discipline themselves to record their observations, hunches–to reflect on them and even dream about them, create a story about whatever they have experienced (the verbatim), and tell that story within their own CPE community. If the story is a "good" one, that is, if the story sits well in the experiences of others, it is accepted as being "true" and may even be passed to future generations until further "truth" is discerned in future stories.

As chaplains we too can pay attention to our work-world in imaginative ways. The argument that set the Baconians over against the imaginings of creative scientists has long misled us and set us up for impoverishment. The good scientist pays attention, and can be at home not just in the realm on the human senses, but in the realms of the spirit and of mental activity. We even have a role model from within our own profession, a chaplain who has greatly influenced us all, Anton Boisen. If chaplains need a role model of someone who was both subject and observer, who scientifically studied himself, we need look no further than he.[18] We do need to be clear about why we engage in research however. Some have argued that we must do research in order to demonstrate that chaplains positively affect a hospital's bottom line, that they bolster the hospital's image in the community, or increase patient/family satisfaction. Unfortunately, whether a hospital has chaplains or not, and how many, appears to depend not on the results of scientific study of any kind, but often on politics and/or personality.

The primary reason for doing research is so that we will be better chaplains, so that we can minister more effectively. The limitations and dangers of traditional science have been well elucidated by Huston Smith in his recent book. He alerts us to it in these words. Believing that science has all the answers "is the kind of misunderstanding of science that got us into the tunnel (of narrowed vision) in the first place, for it belittles art, religion, love and the bulk of the life we directly live by denying that those elements yield insights that are needed to complement what science tells us . . . Our exiting the tunnel requires that science share the knowledge project equitably with other ways of knowing–notably . . . The ways of God-seekers."[19]

It is time to embrace what we are already doing in a weak way, but to do it now deliberately and with resolve, believing that the results will benefit not only our profession, but also the persons to whom we minister. It is time to be fully God-seekers.

NOTES

1. De Chardin T. *Building the Earth*. Translated by Noel Lindsay. Wilkes-Barre, PA: Dimension Books; 1965. The full quotation is: "The time has come to realize that research is the highest human function, embracing the spirit of conflict and bright with the splendor of religion. To keep up a constant pressure on the surface of the real, is not that the supreme gesture (posture) of faith in Being and therefore the highest form of adoration."

2. *Time.* October 22, 1965: 61ff.

3. Mach E. *Die Mechanik in ihrer Entwicklung.* Leipzig, Germany; 1883. Published in English as *The Science of Mechanics.* 1893. Mach is the man who gave us the Mach number for quantifying the speed of high-speed airplanes.

4. See the argument of Polyanyi M. *Personal Knowledge.* Chicago, IL: University of Chicago Press; 1958. Or Barbour I. *Science and Religion.* New York, NY: Harper & Row; 1968, and more recently the extended reflections of Wilbur K. *Sex, Ecology, Spirituality. The Spirit of Evolution.* Boston. MA: Shambhala Press; 1995, especially chapter 7.

5. Quoted by Eslinger R.L. *Narrative and Imagination. Preaching the Worlds That Shape Us.* Minneapolis, MN: Fortress Press; 1995: 68-9.

6. Smith A. The principles which lead and direct philosophical enquiries: illustrated by the history of astronomy. In Wightman W.P.D., Bryce J.C., Ross I.S. (Eds.) *Essays on Philosophical Subjects.* London, Oxford University Press; 1980. 4:III.5. Originally published in 1795 by Davies and Creech. Scotland, Edinburgh.

7. De Chardin, op cit p. 38.

8. This is the reason many of us are concerned that both Christian and Muslim fundamentalists could have the same limiting, even fatal effect in education and science today. The Taliban in Afghanistan and Pakistan had no place for science in their madrassas. The Christian fundamentalists in the US oppose the teaching of evolution.

9. Wilber K. "Eye to eye–Integral philosophy and the quest for the real" in *The Eye of Spirit–An Integral Vision for a World Gone Slightly Mad.* Boston, MA: Shambhala Press; 1998: 84-93. Wilbur accepts the basic structure of the scientific method as it was first suggested by Thomas Kuhn (1970) in *The Structure of the Scientific Revolution.* Chicago, IL: University of Chicago Press. Wilbur describes how the same processes can be found in all three domains of human enquiry: the world we see with our senses; the world see with our inner eye; and, the world of that which does the seeing–the Self. In each of these domains, argues Wilbur, we do what Kuhn has identified in the domain of the senses. First, we follow an instrumental injunction or instruction. Second, we perceive a certain state of affairs. Third, we compare our findings with those of others, the communal confirmation.

10. Glaser B. and Strauss A. *The Discovery of Grounded Theory.* Chicago, IL: Aldine; 1967. An updated description of this method can be found in "Grounded theory research: Procedures, canons, and evaluative criteria" by Corbin J. Strauss A. *Qualitative Sociology* 1990:13(1): 3-21.

11. Macaulay A.A., Commanda L.E., Freeman W.L. et al. in Participatory research maximizes community and lay involvement. *British Medical Journal.* 1999;319(7212): 774-778.

12. Iler W.L., Obenshain D., Camac M., The impact of daily visits from chaplains on patients with chronic obstructive pulmonary disease (COPD): A pilot study. *Chaplaincy Today.* 2001;17(1): 5-11.

13. Kuhn op cit.

14. Wilber op cit pp. 85ff.

15. Friere P. *Pedagogy of the Oppressed.* Translated by Myra Bergman Ramos. New York, NY: Continuum; 1973 (Rev. 1994) and Drane J., Theological education for the next century. *British Journal of Theological Education.* 1995; 6(3): 3-8.

16. Some years after her work with schizophrenics, two seminarians from the University of Chicago Divinity School, Glenn Davidson and Daniel Davis crossed the street to get help for a term paper they were working on. They wanted to talk with someone who was dying, and approached Kubler-Ross, then at the University of Chi-

cago Hospitals. She helped them find a patient, and it was while working with them and in subsequent seminars that she began to wonder if there was any pattern or patterns in the way people did their dying. She described her work with schizophrenics as being the precursor to the model she devised for her understanding of the grief process, in a continuing education seminar for clergy at the University of Michigan Medical Center in the spring of 1974.

17. Corr C.A., Coping with dying: Lessons that we should and should not learn from the work of Elizabeth Ross. *Death Studies.* 1993; 17(1): 69-83.

18. Hart C.W., Notes on the psychiatric diagnosis of Anton Boisen. *Journal of Religion and Health.* 2001; 40(4): 423-429.

19. Smith H. *The Fate of the Human Spirit in the Age of Disbelief.* San Francisco, CA: Harper; 2001. p. 187.

Chaplaincy *Is* Becoming More "Scientific." What's the Problem?

Larry Burton, ThD, BCC

SUMMARY. I argue that chaplaincy does not need to be afraid of research because it is already becoming more scientific. In so doing, it has not lost its soul or identity. It can use research results appropriately to promote the care that is at the heart of its identity. *[Article copies available for a fee from The Haworth Document Delivery Service: 1-800-HAWORTH. E-mail address: <docdelivery@haworthpress.com> Website: <http://www.HaworthPress.com> © 2002 by The Haworth Press, Inc. All rights reserved.]*

KEYWORDS. Chaplaincy, pastoral care, science

"A very interesting report," remarked the VP for Patient Services. "According to these figures, if a patient spends time with one of our chaplains, that patient is more likely to recommend our hospital. Maybe we need to employ chaplain-greeters."

"Very funny," responded the Director of Chaplaincy Services. "You did get the point though. There is something that is going on in the chaplain's visit that increases patient and family satisfaction."

Larry Burton is affiliated with the Gobin Memorial United Methodist Church, 307 Simpson Street, P.O. Box 66, Greencastle, IN 46135 (E-mail: Lburton@CCRTC.com).

[Haworth co-indexing entry note]: "Chaplaincy *Is* Becoming More "Scientific." What's the Problem?" Burton, Larry. Co-published simultaneously in *Journal of Health Care Chaplaincy* (The Haworth Pastoral Press, an imprint of The Haworth Press, Inc.) Vol. 12, No. 1/2, 2002, pp. 43-51; and: *Professional Chaplaincy and Clinical Pastoral Education Should Become More Scientific: Yes and No* (ed: Larry VandeCreek) The Haworth Pastoral Press, an imprint of The Haworth Press, Inc., 2003, pp. 43-51. Single or multiple copies of this article are available for a fee from The Haworth Document Delivery Service [1-800-HAWORTH, 9:00 a.m. - 5:00 p.m. (EST). E-mail address: docdelivery@haworthpress.com].

"Well, it's not just the increase in satisfaction that impresses me. It looks as if when a chaplain works with our patients in rehab, those patients go home faster. This is really good stuff. It's clearer than ever that you chaplains do more than just pray when someone has died. Yes, this is very interesting indeed."

This is a fictional conversation–though there is hardly a chaplain alive who doesn't wish s/he could have this encounter with a hospital executive. Though fictional, it is based on research findings (Fitchett, unpublished; Fitchett, Meyer & Burton, 2000). Such findings are already being used in medical centers to argue for an expansion of chaplaincy services or at least to maintain current services in light of budget cuts.

Yet some people are afraid that such research can (and will!) lead to a fundamental change in chaplaincy. "We are different from the other healthcare professions," goes the argument. "We represent the Transcendent and what we do cannot be quantified. We are not just a commodity to be weighed and measured." At a major chaplaincy meeting several years ago, one of the plenary speakers was a physician with a special interest in chaplaincy. This speaker was presenting an approach to "scientific chaplaincy" that used many of the tools of social science research as well as ideas related to quality improvement. After the presentation–which has been both energetic and spirited–a largely disgruntled audience complained, "That isn't chaplaincy. Chaplaincy is about being present, and you just can't measure that. Those people should just leave chaplains alone."

But chaplains are *not* being left alone. No matter how much some chaplains complain, the profession has already begun to change, and scientific research is part of the change.

RESEARCH AFFECTING CHAPLAINS

Jeff Levin (2001) has said, "It is not over dramatizing things in the least to note that there was a time about fifteen years ago when those of us actively investigating the linkages between religion and health could fit around a single conference table. A very small one" (p. vii-viii). Even that world has changed.

Herbert Benson (1975), having demonstrated the power of the Relaxation Response, went on to wonder about the similarity of that physiological response to the body's response to meditative prayer. In 1997 he reported a variety of benefits ranging from pain control to decreases in sleep-onset insomnia to decreases in hypertension. Other researchers have found positive relationships between religion and health outcomes that have implications for chaplains. The following are only a few examples.

- Hip replacements: Pressman, P., Lyons, J., Larson, D., and Strain, J. 1990. Religious belief, depression, and ambulation status in elderly women with broken hips. *American Journal of Psychiatry*, 147, 758-760.
- Well being among the elderly: Koenig, H., Pargament, K., and Kielsen, J. 1998. Religious coping and health status in medically ill hospitalized older adults. *Journal of Nervous and Mental Disease*, 186, 513-521. Koenig, H., George, L., and Peterson, B. 1998. Religiosity and remission from depression in medically ill older patients. *American Journal of Psychiatry*, 155, 536-542.
- Survival after heart surgery: Oxman, T., Freeman, D., and Manheimer, E. 1995. Lack of social participation or religious strength and comfort as risk factors for death after cardiac surgery in the elderly. *Psychosomatic Medicine*, 57, 5-15.

Levin, himself, has contributed no fewer than 25 studies including studies of attendance at religious services (1987) and the relationship to personal health as well as a model for understanding how prayer heals (1996).

These, and more than a thousand other studies–the majority, but not all, suggesting this positive relationship between religion and health–have been undertaken by physicians, epidemiologists, social scientists, psychologists and chaplains. The methodology ranges from randomized clinical trials to prospective cohort studies to cross-sectional studies. Standard statistical methods are used to control for confounding data, check for measurement error, and generalizability. In short, the field of study conforms to the same criteria as other scientific research. The only difference is, this research involves religion.

THE DEBATE

One would think that the presence of this emerging body of research would be good news to professional chaplains, but that is not necessarily so. Chaplain No whose short piece appears at the beginning of this volume is one of those opposed to chaplaincy "becoming more scientific." This chaplain is concerned because chaplaincy "will not be able to carry out [its] mission as a scientific discipline because science will also define chaplaincy . . ." Even on the face of it, this argument cannot be sustained.

When one thinks of healthcare, medical doctors are the first people that come to mind, followed closely by nursing. Allopathic medicine, perhaps most highly developed in the United States, has gained tremendous power and respect precisely because it has become "more scientific." From Pasteur's introduction of germ theory and Koch's discoveries of the bacterial causes of tuberculosis and cholera (Koenig, McCullough & Larson, 2001), the science of medicine has evolved from rather primitive origins to its current position as near miracle-worker. All the while, the profession of physician, while also evolving, has not changed in terms of its basic mission: to cure when possible and to care always. Nursing has followed a similar path. Why should chaplaincy be different? Precisely because of studies that demonstrate positive correlations between religious beliefs and practices (not all, religious beliefs and practices have a positive correlation it should be noted) there are now chaplains assigned to work in outpatient clinics and physician practices. Chaplains are working on palliative care teams, as part of oncology services, and in EAPs because research demonstrates the effectiveness of helping people assess and access their spiritual resources. Scientific studies have not *defined* chaplaincy, but rather have helped support chaplaincy's self-definition.

BUT WHAT IS IT THAT CHAPLAINS DO, ANYWAY?

Representing the Transcendent in times of crisis is a theological claim with which most professional (and lay!) religious care providers would agree. Indeed, Board Certified Chaplains must be endorsed by their faith group. So chaplains are, by definition, representatives of the Transcendent in one way or another. But the singularity of this claim is problematic. On the one hand a God representative can offer comfort and hope. On the other, this view can be reduced to an image of someone standing at the door of a hospital room and announcing grandly, "Never fear, God's representative is here." While this may be health-ful to some, it may be annoying (at the least) to others. For some it may even be experienced as abusive and unhealthy (Watters, 1992).

I would argue that the contemporary genius of professional chaplaincy is not representing the Transcendent (as important as that is), but rather that chaplains have learned over time–through study and observation and from the scientific research in the field–that each person has her or his own particular spiritual resources that need to be identified, accessed, and supported, especially in times of health crisis. Further, it is also clear from research that some religious beliefs and practices are *not* conducive to health. Koenig et al. (2001) write:

> There is some evidence that religious beliefs that portray God (or a higher power) as distant, uninterested, punishing, or vindictive have less salutary health effects than belief systems that present God as merciful, kind, forgiving, and understanding or as a collaborative partner. In a cross-sectional study of 577 consecutively hospitalized patients age 55 or over, Koenig, Pargament et al., found that appraisals of God as benevolent or as a collaborative partner were related to better mental health. Religious beliefs that viewed God as a punishing deity and demonic forces as responsible for health problems were associated with worse mental health. (p. 70)

Professional chaplains also bring skills in spiritual assessment to help identify potential spiritual risk (Fitchett et al., 2000) and to help patients identify their own spiritual resources for coping and healing. Research (Fitchett, Burton, & Sivan, 1997) has shown that patients can identify spiritual needs, but often do not have a relationship with a spiritual caregiver to help respond to those needs. This is but another example of how scientific research supports and helps focus the work of chaplaincy.

Could science begin to "call the tune" for chaplains? I suppose that could happen. It is possible if there are valid studies indicating, for instance, that effective chaplaincy work could be accomplished in fifteen minutes or less. Then chaplains could come under pressure to produce more patient visits. Anything over fifteen minutes would be scrutinized. But every professional chaplain knows that a traumatic death in the emergency room or a difficult ethics consultation can take hours of a chaplain's time. But there are no such research findings, and the pressure to produce has been present in many institutions for some time, without any foundation other than the managed care imagination.

The important point in this conversation is to remember that "science" does not call the shots, people do. The tail wags the dog only if the dog hasn't done her/his homework.

IS THERE A MORAL OBLIGATION TO IMPROVE?

Those opposed to chaplaincy becoming more scientifically based argue that the profession "is morally obligated to resist this seduction . . ." (refer to chaplain no). This is perhaps an argument grounded in the principle of nonmaleficence (Beauchamp & Childress, 1989), that is "do no harm" (in this case, do no harm to the profession and the professional). On the other side of the aisle is the claim that "chaplaincy is morally obligated to use scientific methods to measure the helpfulness of its practices and to improve them." In contrast to the first principle, this position makes a claim on the principle of beneficence, that is "promote good." When applied to a profession or a professional, it would mean that there is an obligation to help both a profession and its professors to find ways to benefit others. Beauchamp and Childress (1989) write, "Firmly established in the histories of medicine, health care, and public health is the belief that a failure to benefit others–and not simply the failure to avoid harm–in many circumstances violates social or professional or moral obligations" (p. 196).

These claims push the debate into the realm of ethics. The first question then is: Does this qualify as a classic moral dilemma?

Moral dilemmas usually involve a situation when two conflicting courses of action are each morally justified. On the face of it the claim that chaplaincy should always be ready and willing to improve the delivery of its services seems perfectly logical and correct. Isn't the goal of chaplaincy "healing through spiritual care?" The spiritual (related to the physical) well-being of patients is the primary concern of the chaplain. Why would any profession so oriented contend that it should *not* be concerned about the improving its services? Would we want to go to a physician who proudly advertised that s/he hadn't altered her/his practice in light of scientific discoveries? Of course not. In fact, most board certified doctors (and board certified chaplains!) must engage in continuing education precisely because of the commitment to maintaining quality and improving practice. Here one avoids doing harm and seeks to do good by grounding practice in sound research findings.

On the other hand, good scientists know that there is no such thing as value free science. Research can be used to promote questionable agendas (Annas & Grodin, 1992). It would be naïve to think that just because a study claims to prove this or that thing, that chaplains, as a profession, are morally obligated to practice it in the name of improvement. When Randolph Byrd (1988), a cardiologist in San Francisco, published an article claiming "proof positive" evidence for the healing power of intercessory prayer, most scientists did not know what to do with the findings. The results were attacked on methodological grounds (that debate continues) or dismissed as an attempt to "prove God." However, some delighted in the findings. What if, based on Byrd's study, chaplains were required by hospital administrators to engage in intercessory prayer for all CABG patients with the intent to reduce the length of stay and therefore save important healthcare dollars? While some would find this perfectly natural ("I pray for my patients no matter what"), others would worry about praying for patients of different religious traditions, or praying for someone without their permission ("If prayer is that effective, it is a treatment, and it just isn't right to treat people without their consent"). Most chaplains would agree that, no matter how well intended, to engage in a practice–even a routine visit–without a patient's consent would (or at least could) cause harm and would therefore be avoided. In this context the question is, does relying on scientific research harm the profession of chaplaincy, and thereby harm patients?

The issue of how chaplaincy should relate to scientific studies is not "either/or." Chaplains do not have to accept every study that comes down the pike in order to improve practice. Nor do they have to reject the results of research simply because they are afraid of losing control of our profession.

So, do we have a moral dilemma? I don't think so. While chaplains, like all professionals, must keep a keen eye out for self-deception ("Come on, what's your problem? There's no real issue here and it might do some good") one is hard pressed to find a moral duty to oppose the professional application of scientific findings in the service of patient health and well-being. If there is a moral duty, it is to promote the good of our patients without falling into the trap of paternalism (Beauchamp & Childress, 1989).

ONE FINAL QUESTION

There is still one question left. The original question (Should professional chaplaincy become more scientific?) added a final phrase: "in response to health care reform." Here, of course, the key is one's understanding of health care reform. One suspects that the idea of reforming healthcare, based in the 1990s response to escalating health care costs and culminating in the many manifestations of managed care, has waned. While it is true that some hospitals are still undergoing the process of become "mean and lean" (a phrase that is particularly repugnant to anyone in a caring profession), that is not the current climate.

Though healthcare costs, as a portion of the Gross Domestic Product, are climbing again, spending more than 1.4 trillion dollars annually or 14 percent of the GDP (Gigs Information Group, 2001), it is unlikely that we will see the same response we saw five and ten years ago. In fact, I want to make a different kind of suggestion about chaplaincy and health care reform.

This is the time for professional chaplains (and all others concerned about the relationship of spirituality, religion and health) to take the lead. If there is to be a new wave of reform, it is likely to be more evidence-based. That is, decisions about interventions and staffing will be founded, as much as possible, on scientific research. Currently, even hospitals sponsored by religious groups are not necessarily leaders in providing spiritual care. It is not that they don't think it matters, it is just that they have only their intuition or their faith to go on, and that doesn't always justify the expense. Chaplaincy *does* make a significant contribution to healthcare whether in a direct manner or in a value-added way (VandeCreek & Burton, 2001). Chaplains need to be actors, not those who are acted upon.

Chaplaincy is already becoming more scientific. That has not meant a loss of heart or a loss of identity. We do not have to be afraid of research. Rather we can use the findings of research appropriately to promote the care that is at the heart of our identity.

REFERENCES

Annas, G. and Grodin, M. (1992). *The Nazi Doctors and the Nuremberg Code: Human Rights in Human Experimentation*. NY: Oxford University Press.

Beauchamp, T. and Childress, J. (1989). *Principles of Biomedical Ethics*. NY: Oxford University Press.

Benson, H. (1975). *The Relaxation Response*. NY: William Morrow.

Benson, H. (1997). *Timeless Healing*. NY: Simon and Schuster.

Byrd, R. (1988). Positive therapeutic effects of intercessory prayer in a coronary care unit population. *Southern Medical Journal*, 81, 826-829.

Fitchett, G., Burton, L., and Sivan, A. (1997). The religious needs and resources of psychiatric patients. *Journal of Nervous and Mental Disease*, 185, 320-326.

Fitchett, G., Meyer, P., and Burton L. (2000). Spiritual care in the hospital: Who requests it? Who needs it? *Journal of Pastoral Care* 54(2), 173-186.

Fitchett, G. Unpublished patient satisfaction studies, Rush-Presbyterian-St. Luke's Medical Center, Chicago, IL.

Giga Information Group, 5/31/2001.

Koenig, H., McCullough, M., and Larson, D. (2001). *Handbook of Religion and Health.* NY: Oxford University Press.

Levin, J. and Vanderpool, H. (1987). Is frequent religious attendance really conducive to better health? Toward an epidemiology of religion. *Social Science and Medicine*, 24, 589-600.

Levin, J. (1996). How prayer heals: A theoretical model. *Alternative Therapies*, 2(1), 66-73.

Levin, J. (2001). "Forward" in Koenig, H., McCullough, M., and Larson, D. *Handbook of Religion and Health.* NY: Oxford University Press.

VandeCreek, L. and Burton, L. (ed). (2001). *Processional Chaplaincy: Its Role and Importance in Healthcare.* Published by ACPE, APC, CAPPE, NACC and NAJC.

Watters, W. (1992). *Deadly Doctrine: Health, Illness, and Christian God-Talk.* Buffalo, NY: Prometheus.

Clinical Pastoral Education and the Value of Empirical Research: Examples from Australian and New Zealand Datum

Rev. Chap. Lindsay B. Carey, MAppSc, RAAF
Rev. Dr. Christopher Newell, AM, PhD

SUMMARY. This article argues in favor of clinical pastoral education programs incorporating research methods as part of a standard neo-curriculum for the 21st Century. It suggests that the benefits of such a curriculum would be useful in scientifically validating and evaluating pastoral care practice at a 'micro,' 'meso' and 'macro' level. This argument is supported with the presentation of Australian and New Zealand descriptive statistical datum exploring the involvement of chaplains in patient bioethical decisions, staff bioethical decision-making and the involvement of chaplains on hospital institutional research ethics committees.

Rev. Chap. Lindsay B. Carey is National Research Officer, Australian Health & Welfare Chaplains Association, School of Public Health, La Trobe University, Victoria, Australia (E-mail: Linz.Carey@latrobe.edu.au). Rev. Dr. Christopher Newell is Consultant Ethicist and Senior Lecturer, School of Medicine, University of Tasmania, Hobart, Australia (E-mail: Christopher.Newell@utas.edu.au).

[Haworth co-indexing entry note]: "Clinical Pastoral Education and the Value of Empirical Research: Examples from Australian and New Zealand Datum." Carey, Lindsay B. and Christopher Newell. Co-published simultaneously in *Journal of Health Care Chaplaincy* (The Haworth Pastoral Press, an imprint of The Haworth Press, Inc.) Vol. 12, No. 1/2, 2002, pp. 53-65; and: *Professional Chaplaincy and Clinical Pastoral Education Should Become More Scientific: Yes and No* (ed: Larry VandeCreek) The Haworth Pastoral Press, an imprint of The Haworth Press, Inc., 2003, pp. 53-65. Single or multiple copies of this article are available for a fee from The Haworth Document Delivery Service [1-800-HAWORTH, 9:00 a.m. - 5:00 p.m. (EST). E-mail address: docdelivery@haworthpress.com].

[Article copies available for a fee from The Haworth Document Delivery Service: 1-800-HAWORTH. E-mail address: <docdelivery@haworthpress.com> Website: <http://www.HaworthPress.com> © 2002 by The Haworth Press, Inc. All rights reserved.]

KEYWORDS. Clinical pastoral education, chaplaincy, science, research

. . . we have not built an empirical research tradition that tests our observations and theories . . . That, I believe, makes us morally culpable. As members of our respective organizations we have been too ready to make a living on existing, borrowed insights and practice patterns, and not ready enough to test our own insights. Consequently, we can legitimately been seen in the scientific world as a "do nothing" profession which has failed to make a contribution to knowledge in a scientific age. (VandeCreek, 1988, p. 2-3)

In this article we suggest that VandeCreek's (1988) critique of pastoral care is current to Australian and New Zealand (ANZ) Clinical Pastoral Education (CPE). Without an adequate research basis it can be argued that CPE, and pastoral care in general, will be largely dismissed as an insignificant discipline within ANZ's future contemporary health care. Admittedly some empirical research, undertaken within Australian medical settings, has indicated that medical, nursing and allied health staff largely approve of the role and work of pastoral carers and chaplains in regard to their 'support' of patient and staff well-being (Carey et al., 1997). Yet pastoral carers and chaplains are often perceived as *not* having a 'serious' clinical disciplinary basis for practice. Indeed, because of past and current scientific-anti-religious-perspectives, pastoral care is consequently viewed in the wider health arena as somewhat of an anachronism. Unfortunately, in a world of evidence-based care, many CPE supervisors continue to teach CPE largely without incorporating any research skills to aid critical reflection and evaluation of practice. Consequently ANZ chaplains have largely based their practice upon pastoral care techniques that have little research base. Thus the majority of CPE graduates emerge and will continue to emerge without a culture of research, untrained to critically investigate their own practice, and without sufficient ability to create pastoral care that is evidence-based.

Such a state of affairs would seem to 'fly in the face' of early contributors to CPE such as William S. Keller, Joseph Fletcher, Richard C. Cabot and Anton Boisen, who sought through CPE to ensure that 'religion might be more relevant to the lives of persons in crisis.' In the past this has been achieved by the CPE educational techniques of 'experience,' 'reflection,' 'insight,' 'action and integration' (Cotterell & Nisi, 1990, p. 138). However it seems timely to include 'research and evaluation' which can also ensure that these afore-mentioned dimensions of CPE are used in the best possible educational way.

CPE: A CRITICAL EVALUATION

Like all professional and educational programs CPE has and can be criticized on many fronts. On the Australian front, such criticisms have included a lack of critical reflection on power relations, lack of uniform quality assurance, significant under-explored ethical issues in supervision and group work, and a lack of research concerning the impact and experience of CPE upon students. It has even been suggested that pastoral carers have opportunities to identify a variety of systemic issues but little in the way of conceptual tools to assess such issues (i.e., research skills) (Newell, 1997).

Further, as Hemenway (1996) paraphrases Ahlskog (1993), there is the '. . . inherent weakness of process education (CPE) in which "student centered learning" not only ignores conceptual knowledge but also presumes that to claim personal growth in self-knowledge, self-authentication and self-direction is sufficient to receive skills for doing ministry.' Increasingly one of the crucial skills for those undertaking ministry training under the CPE model is to be able to establish themselves as professionals who have something to contribute towards better health care than simply advocating religious or ecclesiastical platitudes. In our experience, in the Australasian clinical scene, it seems that good pastoral care counselling skills are no longer solely sufficient when planning clinical pathways.

Perhaps the most serious criticism of CPE is the lack of empirical research training. VandeCreek et al. (1994) has noted several classical concerns as to why clergy are reluctant to facilitate pastoral care research. Namely, (i) that the 'personalities of clergy' tend be caring, intuitive and supportive with emphasis upon faith and hope rather than scientific skepticism; (ii) that the 'theological-educational focus' of training ministers does not usually involve science and mathematical-statistical research and thus it is seemingly not ratified by ecclesiastical institutions as appropriate for clergy to focus upon or engage in such studies; (iii) that clergy develop a theologically-philosophically based 'ministry focus' which seems to conflict with the arenas of science and scientific methods.

While these concerns are legitimate issues, such concerns do not provide sufficient argument against evaluation methods appropriate to the clinical environment. As people who have benefited from CPE (in various ways) we acknowledge that there is much that is good about CPE and that CPE should, like other clinical disciplines, be a combination of *both* art and science. Yet as practicing researchers we have become extremely concerned, at not only the lack of ANZ scientific research with regard to CPE and pastoral care, but also a culture within CPE that is almost hostile to scientific research. This attitude may cause a challenge to the credentialing and practice of ANZ CPE in the future. We suggest that research methods, incorporated into CPE training, should not simply be implemented to convince scientists and health care administrators that pastoral care services are important to maintain, but such a move can help to provide empirical evidence to guide the future direction of CPE courses and benefit the training and work of CPE supervisors.

In our experience, CPE supervisors in ANZ are clearly professionally skilled and valued practitioners but we have little evidence for that and little evidence to support the funding of CPE programs in ANZ institutions in a world of tightening hospital and church budgets–both of which have become subject to varying degrees of economic rationalism and downsizing (VandeCreek, 2000; Newell & Carey, 2000). In Australia whilst there is a requirement for CPE supervisors to write papers, as part of gaining their supervisory credential, this does not necessarily equip them to critically evaluate research and to conduct research. More importantly most CPE supervisory training does not have research methods instruction for CPE students so that a new culture of ANZ pastoral care may be fostered–where research is the norm (rather than the exception) and pastoral care clinical practice has a research justification which is substantial, readily accessible and becomes well known to associated professionals.

CPE: RESEARCH AT THE MICRO-LEVEL

At this point it is important that we 'practice what we preach' and consider Australian and New Zealand datum comparing chaplains who have completed CPE and those who have no CPE training and their involvement in bioethical issues. It is not possible to provide in depth analysis and discussion within this paper about the issues raised by the following research results. Rather the following basic descriptive statistical results are presented in order to raise numerous and pertinent questions that highlight the need for CPE to incorporate research protocols.

The 'Australian and New Zealand Chaplaincy Utility Research' study (ANZ.CUR), which has been exploring the issues of pastoral care and bioethics, involved over 327 members of the Australian Health & Welfare Chaplains Association. Within New Zealand (NZ) duplicate research involved 100 health care chaplaincy personnel, working under the auspices of the NZ ICCHC (Inter-Church Council on Hospital Chaplaincy). This research indicated that the majority of Australian health care (stipended) chaplains (76.2%) and non-stipended 'volunteer chaplains' (52.3%) completed at least one unit of CPE (Figure 1). The results also indicated that the majority of NZ health care stipended chaplains (75.4%) and a minority of volunteer non-stipended 'assistant chaplains' (30.2%) had completed at least one unit of CPE (Figure 1).

Such percentages of chaplains completing CPE should be seen as a credit to both the AHWCA and the ICHC for promoting clinical pastoral education and chaplaincy employment standards beyond the basics of minimal ecclesiastical knowledge for both stipended and voluntary chaplains. Yet such results also raise some questions that require further consideration.

The question must be asked: 'What of those ANZ chaplains (whether stipended or volunteers) who had not completed CPE?' (AU 26%; NZ

FIGURE 1. Chaplains and Volunteer Chaplains (Australia [AU n = 327] and New Zealand [NZ n = 100]) by completion or no completion of CPE.

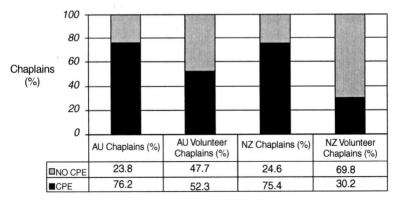

	AU Chaplains (%)	AU Volunteer Chaplains (%)	NZ Chaplains (%)	NZ Volunteer Chaplains (%)
▫ NO CPE	23.8	47.7	24.6	69.8
▪ CPE	76.2	52.3	75.4	30.2

35.5%). 'What standards and quality of service did they offer to patients and their families at the bedside?' These questions raise issues that should not be muted. Such questions should particularly be asked when one considers that the ANZ.CUR study also revealed that a majority of Australian health care chaplains (83.8%) and volunteer chaplains (52.8%) had been involved in assisting patients (or their families) to make decisions concerning one or more critical bioethical issues (e.g., pain control, withdrawal of life support, DNR orders). Of those involved in assisting with patient bioethical decisions, one fifth (20.18%) of Australian chaplains and volunteer chaplains had *no* CPE training. Likewise, among New Zealand chaplaincy personnel, of those involved in assisting patients (or their families) to make critical bioethical decisions, 15.7% of NZ chaplains and 13.9% of NZ volunteer chaplains had *no* CPE training (refer Figure 2).

The results of such research raise challenging questions such as, 'What methodology and techniques are *non*-CPE trained chaplains using during critical bio-ethical decision making?' and 'What are the outcomes of methods used by non-CPE trained chaplaincy personnel in comparison to CPE trained chaplaincy personnel?' Further, 'By what methods do pastoral care departments/ supervisors hold their *non*-CPE trained chaplains accountable?'

FIGURE 2. Chaplains and Volunteer Chaplains (Australia [AU n = 327] and New Zealand [NZ n = 100]) by CPE training and involvement in PATIENT bioethical decisions.

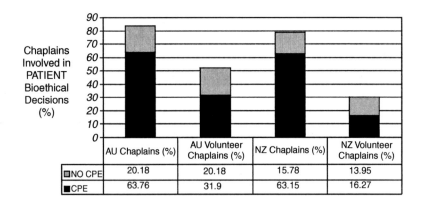

	AU Chaplains (%)	AU Volunteer Chaplains (%)	NZ Chaplains (%)	NZ Volunteer Chaplains (%)
□NO CPE	20.18	20.18	15.78	13.95
■CPE	63.76	31.9	63.15	16.27

We may also here reflect that there is a prior question to ascertain: 'Is CPE the most effective method to train and sustain pastoral cares/chaplains in preparation for critical patient bioethical dilemmas?' Such questions cannot be asked or argued continuously at the philosophical or theological level. CPE itself needs to be tested in terms of 'patient benefit effectiveness.' Systematic and empirical research is required. Indeed, if clinical pastoral education is to maintain the term 'clinical' one could well argue that, like all professional occupations, a scientific approach to qualify methods and to achieve improved quality assurance is required.

CPE: RESEARCH AT THE MESO-LEVEL

It is a common assumption made by some people that a chaplain exclusively serves the needs of patients and their families. The contribution that chaplains and their respective departments make in terms of assisting staff with complex bioethical issues at ward, unit or departmental level is often overlooked. The ANZ.CUR study indicated that approximately 58% of Australian chaplains and 25% of Australian volunteer chaplains were involved in assisting clinical staff with bioethical decisions. Among New Zealand respondents, 48% of NZ Chaplains and 16% of NZ Volunteer chaplains assisted staff with bioethical decisions. Of these, approximately between 9-14% of Australian chaplaincy personnel had no CPE training and between 3-9% of NZ chaplaincy personnel had no CPE training (refer Figure 3).

Again practical questions need to be addressed: 'What methodology and information have non-CPE chaplains used to assist and/or advise clinical staff and their respective wards, units or departments about bioethical issues?' 'How have pastoral care departments assessed the contribution which chaplains make to wards, units or other departments?' Indeed, 'How have other departments and their staff perceived the utility of chaplains?' and of 'What professional and/or personal importance have staff placed upon the role and work of chaplains and their respective pastoral care departments?' The present authors argue that such questions raise the need for research and for chaplains to be trained in research methods to conduct and/or evaluate pastoral care practice.

FIGURE 3. Chaplains and Volunteer Chaplains (Australia [AU n = 327] and New Zealand [NZ n = 100]) by CPE training and involvement in STAFF bioethical decisions.

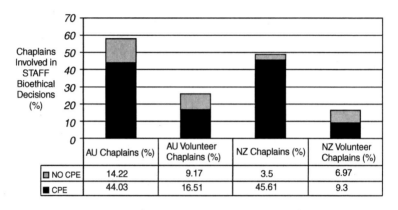

	AU Chaplains (%)	AU Volunteer Chaplains (%)	NZ Chaplains (%)	NZ Volunteer Chaplains (%)
NO CPE	14.22	9.17	3.5	6.97
CPE	44.03	16.51	45.61	9.3

CPE: RESEARCH AT THE MACRO-LEVEL

A role that is sometimes undertaken by ministers of religion and chaplains at a macro-institutional level is that of being a member of a Human Research Ethics Committee (HREC), previously termed hospital ethics committees. This is particularly the case in Australia where it has become a mandatory expectation of the *National Statement on Ethical Conduct in Research Involving Humans* published by the National Health and Medical Research Council (1999) that a HREC should include a 'minister of religion' or equivalent as, '. . . ministers of religion are widely seen in our society to be privy to the thoughts and concerns of many people from different back-grounds' (NHMRC, 1985). Results of the ANZ.CUR research indicated that 88.9% of Australian chaplaincy personnel and 30% of New Zealand chaplaincy personnel believed that chaplains should be involved in the decision-making processes of hospital ethics committees. Interestingly, at the time of the research, only 22.3% of Australian chaplaincy personnel and only 8% of New Zealand chaplaincy personnel indicated any actual involvement (refer Figure 4).

Quantitative and qualitative research involving 42 Australian research ethics committees conducted by McNeill et al. (1996) indicated that ministers of religion on hospital ethics committees (the majority of whom were chaplains) were, similar to lay members, '. . . usually perceived to be relatively inactive, and their views were seen to be rela-

FIGURE 4. Percentage of Australian (AU n = 327) and New Zealand (NZ n = 100) Chaplaincy Personnel who believe that chaplains should be involved in the decision making process of Hospital Research Ethics Committees compared with the percentage of AU and NZ chaplains actually involved in HREC decisions.

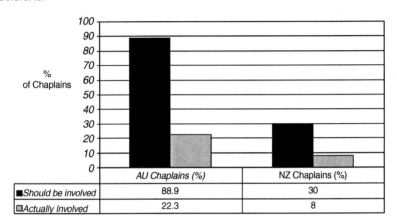

	AU Chaplains (%)	NZ Chaplains (%)
■ Should be involved	88.9	30
☐ Actually Involved	22.3	8

tively unimportant.' One of the main reasons for this perception by other ethics committee members was due to the chaplain's 'lack of expertise.' One chaplain informant noted that, in any HEC decision, he [the chaplain] was '. . . always convinced by the medical argument that the research had to be done' (McNeil et al., 1996, p. 21, 23).

Arguments favoring clergy on HECs have included that, ministers of religion/chaplains have '. . . experience of working within ideologically diverse environments' and '. . . experience in applying principles to real life situations in a dynamic way' plus an '. . . awareness of the limitations of rule-based systems' (McIver, 1996). Yet as Muschamp argues a 'school teacher' could easily substitute for a minister of religion based on such arguments (Muschamp, 1996).

The question arises then, 'What makes the contribution of chaplaincy unique from other 'helping' professions such as social workers, psychologists and even teachers?' Such a question warrants another research project that is currently being worked on by the ANZ.CUR research team. However, in brief, we would argue that, there are two important reasons for having chaplains on HECs. First, the practical experience of chaplains 'working the wards' and being involved in patient and staff bioethical decisions, on an almost daily basis, gives chaplains a unique and regular insight and, combined with their theological and ethical training, a valuable wisdom and pastoral discernment that can assist patients, their families and staff with difficult decision making. Second, the primary values bias of the work of mainstream ministers of religion is that of the dignity–the inherent worth of the human person. In short, people are absolutely important which is what often motivates chaplains to work in the clinical environment.

Against McNeil et al. (1996) and Muschamp's (1996) argument (making the case for the exclusion of chaplains from ethics committees) we would suggest that the rationale for ministers of religion/chaplains being involved on such committees is by virtue of their regular clinical pastoral experience and their primary focus being advocacy for the dignity and welfare of patient/family participants. Clearly however, given that ecclesiastical training and CPE does not include training in research methods, ministers of religion/chaplains are not adequately prepared to deal with the additional demands engaged in a clinical research culture. This is undoubtedly a factor behind the reluctance of some ethics committees to ask chaplains to assist them with committee decisions and a reluctance of chaplains to participate on ethics committees. Yet all other professional representatives on human research ethics committees have received research method training as an integral part of their professional development. Certainly a mix of scientific training with religious ethics could make for chaplains a powerful contribution to any ethics committee.

CPE: ISSUES OF THE FUTURE

It can be argued that there is a need for CPE to undertake research at three levels. At the micro level clinical pastoral education and its educators need to evaluate CPE methodology and techniques in regard to the care of patients and their families. If CPE, empirically measured, *is* found to be effective, particularly in terms of enhancing the well being of patients and their families, then there is a need to be concerned about any chaplain who has *not* undertaken CPE training. If, on the other hand, CPE is found to be ineffective, then, as currently constituted, it is a superfluous program.

At the meso-level, research could be done within hospitals to determine whether clinical pastoral education is benefiting the work of clinical staff, their unit and/or departments. Research on the effectiveness and efficiency of CPE, as a form of quality assurance for a pastoral care departments might, in turn, maximize opportunities for departmental growth and improve the quality of services being offered through the hospital to the community. Likewise, at the macro level, training in research methodology, that would enable a chaplain to be more effective in understanding research protocols, would benefit the hospital as an institution. This could, particularly, be in terms of chaplains being more productive on hospital ethics committees but also in terms of chaplains developing and conducting their own research to benefit the pastoral care services of health care institutions.

Of course, we need to acknowledge the two dimensions of research crucial to the development of CPE as an effective mode of education. Scientific research with its focus on empirical fact, often referred to as quantitative research, is clearly crucial. Yet qualitative research, with its focus on personal narrative and subjective experience, also has an important role. ANZ pastoral research requires CPE graduates to undertake training in both areas as often a particular research question may well need to be tackled by one or the other, or more innovatively, a combination of the two techniques. In our experience pastoral research is more likely to be effective if the qualitative component rests upon a quantitative analysis.

It is of course important to acknowledge that the change required of CPE in ANZ may require skills that some current supervisors do not have. Here we would suggest that a coalition with other research trained health professionals, sympathetic to CPE, is important. Indeed Newell has argued for a vision of Australian CPE supervision that has leadership within mainstream clinical schools that draws upon inter-disciplinary competence (Newell, 1997). It may also be important to identify and locate those clergy who have, at some stage in their career/s, completed training in research methodology. Such skills need to be rekindled and fostered for the betterment of pastoral care services.

It is also important to acknowledge that there are some examples of research projects being undertaken by some ANZ chaplains that have commenced to gather quantitative and/or qualitative data using clinical research techniques (e.g., Ireland, Carey et al., 1998; Gibbons, 1998; Manks, 2002; Davoren, 2002). We would also recognize that there are models of supervision and group work similar to CPE, such as practiced in parts of the United Kingdom, with research competent chaplains. The ANZ CPE lack of research base is such that we are not able to compare such approaches across national boundaries, making a further case for standard educational practices of pastoral carers that are evidence-based.

Finally while it might be argued that having an effective CPE training program that incorporates research methodology provides benefits at micro, meso and macro levels, it does not of course provide certainty against the effects of economic rationalism (Newell & Carey, 2000) or downsizing (VandeCreek, 2000) of pastoral care departments. Nevertheless such uncertainty should not lead to indifference about having a systematic method of evaluating CPE and the procedures for training in such methods. Indeed not to do so is to equate CPE beyond reproach–a status that the majority of clinically trained 'Aussie' and 'Kiwi' professionals will not tolerate indefinitely.

CPE in Australia and New Zealand; Will it survive and thrive to the end of the 21st Century? We would suggest that in order for CPE to thrive effectively and efficiently into the future it can only do so from a firm and ongoing research base.

REFERENCES

Ahlskog, G. (1992) They had to beg us to pray: Reflections on the undesirability of clinical pastoral education. *The Journal of Pastoral Care.* 2 (Summer): p. 179-87.

Carey, L.B., Aroni, R., & Edwards, A. (1997) Health & well being: Hospital chaplaincy, *Health Policy in Australia*, Oxford University Press, Melbourne, p. 190-210.

Carey, L.B. (1997) The role of chaplains: A research overview, *Journal of Health Care Chaplaincy*, [Cambridge], Vol. 9, No. 2, p. 41-53.

Carey, L.B., Aroni, R., Edwards, A.R., Carey-Sargeant, C.L. & Boer, J. (1997) Speech Pathology Practice: Speech pathology and the role of chaplains, *Australian Communication Quarterly*, Autumn, 38-41.

Carey, L.B. (2000) Clinical perspectives on the chaplains prayer role, *Ministry, Society & Theology*, [Melbourne] Vol. 14, No. 1, p. 45-72.

Carey, L.B., Aroni, R., & Gronlund, M. (2000) Biomedical ethics, clinical decision making and hospital chaplaincy in New Zealand, *Ministry, Society & Theology*, [Melbourne], Vol. 12, No. 2, p. 136-156.

Carey, L.B., Aroni, R., & Newell, C. (2002) Pastoral Care & Bioethics: The role of Australian & New Zealand Chaplains in clinical decision making, Australian Chaplaincy Utility Research [Research in progress].

Cotterell, D., & Nisis, W.F. (1990) Clinical Pastoral Education, In: Hayes, H. & Van der Poel, C.J., *Health Care Ministry: A handbook for chaplains*, National Association of Catholic Chaplains, Paulist Press, New York.

Davoren, R. (2002) 'Interfaith Ministry and Hospital Chaplaincy,' Master of Ministry Thesis, Melbourne College of Divinity, Kew, Victoria [Research in progress].

Edwards, N. (1999) Sonnet on the passing of CPE, Ministry, Society & Theology, Vol. 13, No.1, p. 118.

Elliot, H. & Carey, L.B. (1996) The hospital chaplains role in an organ transplant unit, *Ministry, Society & Theology*, [Melbourne], Vol. 10, No. 1, p. 66-78.

Gibbons, G. D. (1996) Pastoral care casemix codings: An attempt to integrate theology, clinical pastoral education and hospital ministry traditions with recent developments in information technology, *Ministry, Society & Theology*, [Melbourne], Vol. 10, No. 1, p. 44-65.

Hemenway, J.E. (1996) *Inside the circle*, Journal of Pastoral Care Publications, Decatur, Georgia.

Ireland, B., Carey, L.B., Baguley, I., Maurizi, R., Crooks, J., & Gronlund, M. (1999) The Westmead Hospital Brain Injury Rehabilitation Unit & Pastoral Care Department pilot research project: A joint research endeavour, *Ministry, Society & Theology*, Vol. 13, No. 1, p. 46-60.

Manks, D. (2002) Introducing Clinical Pastoral Education to Barwon Health: What difference does it make?, Master of Ministry Thesis, Melbourne College of Divinity, Kew, Victoria, Australia [In progress].

McIver, R. K. (1996) Should ministers of religion be on hospital ethics committees?, *Monash Bioethics Review*, Vol. 15, No. 3, p. 14-17.

McNeill, P.M., Berglund, C., & Webster, I.W. (1996) How much influence do various members have within research ethics committees?, *Monash Bioethics Review*, July, Vol. 15, No. 2, p. 16-26.

Muschamp, D. (1996) A rejoinder to McIver, *Monash Bioethics Review*, Vol. 15, No. 3, p. 18-19.

Newell, C. & Carey, L.B. (2000) Economic rationalism and the cost efficiency of hospital chaplaincy, *Journal of Health Care Chaplaincy*, Vol. 10, No. 1, p. 31-52.

Newell, C. (1997) 'Pastoral Care and Ethics: Some Reflections,' *Ministry, Society and Theology*, Vol. 11, No. 2, November, pp. 102-113.

National Health & Medical Research Council (NH&MRC) (1985) *National Health & Medical Research Council Guidelines on Hospital Research Ethics Committees*, Australian Government Publications, Canberra.

NH&MRC (1999) *National Statement on Ethical Conduct in Research Involving Humans*, National Health and Medical Research Council, Canberra.

VandeCreek, L. (2000) How has health care reform affected professional chaplaincy programs and how are department directors responding? *Journal of Health Care Chaplaincy*, Vol. 10, No. 1, p. 7-17.

VandeCreek, L., Bender, H., & Jordan, M.R. (1994) *Research in pastoral care and counselling: Quantitative and qualitative approaches*, Journal of Pastoral Care Publications, Inc., Decatur, Georgia.

VandeCreek, L. (1988) *A research primer for pastoral care and counseling*, Journal of Pastoral Care and Counseling, Decatur, Georgia, p. 3.

Health Care Chaplaincy as a Research-Informed Profession: How We Get There

George Fitchett, DMin, BCC

SUMMARY. Health care chaplaincy should become a research-informed profession in the next ten years. This article describes my rationale for this statement and outlines a plan for accomplishing it. This means that all professional health care chaplains will value the contributions that research can make to their ministry and some chaplains will be engaged in research that informs the profession. Becoming a research-informed profession does not mean losing our emphasis on compassion, faith, presence, self-awareness, or any of the other rich resources of our tradition. It does mean supplementing those resources with the information research provides. I conclude that the question that professional health care chaplains face is not whether to become a research-informed profession, but how to get there. *[Article copies available for a fee from The Haworth Document Delivery Service: 1-800-HAWORTH. E-mail address: <docdelivery@haworthpress.com> Website: <http://www.HaworthPress.com> © 2002 by The Haworth Press, Inc. All rights reserved.]*

KEYWORDS. Chaplaincy, pastoral care, research, science

George Fitchett is Associate Professor and Director of Research, Department of Religion, Health, and Human Values, Rush-Presbyterian-St. Luke's Medical Center, Chicago, IL (E-mail: George_Fitchett@rush.edu).

[Haworth co-indexing entry note]: "Health Care Chaplaincy as a Research-Informed Profession: How We Get There." Fitchett, George. Co-published simultaneously in *Journal of Health Care Chaplaincy* (The Haworth Pastoral Press, an imprint of The Haworth Press, Inc.) Vol. 12, No. 1/2, 2002, pp. 67-72; and: *Professional Chaplaincy and Clinical Pastoral Education Should Become More Scientific: Yes and No* (ed: Larry VandeCreek) The Haworth Pastoral Press, an imprint of The Haworth Press, Inc., 2003, pp. 67-72. Single or multiple copies of this article are available for a fee from The Haworth Document Delivery Service [1-800-HAWORTH, 9:00 a.m. - 5:00 p.m. (EST). E-mail address: docdelivery@haworthpress.com].

10.1300/J080v12n01_07

Health care chaplaincy should become a research-informed profession in the next 10 years. The strategy to accomplish this as I describe it here is directed toward the Association of Professional Chaplains (APC), its leaders and members. I have directed the strategy towards APC for two reasons. First, it is the largest interfaith association of professional chaplains. Second, it is the professional chaplaincy organization that I know best and in which I hold membership. However, in focusing on the APC, I do not wish to exclude the National Association of Catholics Chaplains (NACC), the National Association of Jewish Chaplains (NAJC), nor the Association for Clinical Pastoral Education (ACPE). I hope that the leaders and members of each of these organizations, and those of other interested cognate groups, will also adopt this strategy with whatever modifications are appropriate for their respective organizations.

THE RATIONALE FOR RESEARCH

I briefly suggest three important reasons for integrating research into our profession: it will strengthen our practice of ministry; increase awareness of what we contribute; and promote interdisciplinary relationships. Research can strengthen our ministry in many ways. For example, building on the work of others, my own research (Fitchett, 1999a; 1999b; Fitchett et al., 2000) has examined the contribution of spiritual risk to poor recovery or adjustment of patients. Using this research, chaplains can design referral systems that will help them make better use of their time and be more intentional and effective in their pastoral conversations with patients who show signs of spiritual risk. We all struggle with how to communicate the contribution our ministry makes to the patients, families, and institutions. Research, such as Iler's (2002) work concerning ministry to pulmonary patient, or the research of VandeCreek and Lyon (1997) on patient satisfaction, is an effective way to document the contribution of our ministry. Research collaboration with health care colleagues strengthens our relationships as we integrate research into our professional practice.

TEN-YEAR GOALS

The issue facing professional health care chaplains is not whether but how to become a research-informed profession. In order to achieve this goal, APC should adopt the following as one of its top 3 goals for each of the next 10 years:

> By 2011 all board certified chaplains will value research, be research literate and some members will regularly conduct research.

To achieve this goal, incremental steps are necessary. Identifying outcomes will help us measure our progress. I propose the following steps.

Step 1: Valuing Research for Effective Ministry. In the next 5 years, 100 percent of APC board certified chaplains will value research in general. Evidence for completing this step includes the ability of certified chaplains to identify one well-conducted piece of published research and to describe its relevance for their ministry.

Step 2: Becoming Research Literate. In the next 5 years, 50% of the membership of APC will become research literate, and in the next 10 years, 100% of the membership will be research literate. The evidence for research literacy will include valuing research as described above. In addition, for each chaplain, research literacy will include: (1) Being able to describe the basic elements of good qualitative and quantitative research. (2) Being able to identify specific publications sources where quality research concerning ministry is found. (3) Reading several new research articles related to their ministry each year.

Step 3: Doing Research. In the next 10 years some chaplains will do research as part of their regular job description. To reach this goal, I suggest that approximately 1 percent of our members (about 30 chaplains) become active researcher in 5 years and 2 percent (about 60 chaplains) in 10 years. The evidence for reaching this goal includes both research collaboration with others (being a co-investigator) and leadership in conducting research (being the principal investigator).

Implementing the Goals Achieving these goals must be the work of all APC leaders and members, not just a few people on the research committee. Achieving these goals will require significant educational efforts, changes in certification and continuing education policies, and coordination. By making a commitment to become a research-informed profession, APC may also be able to attract additional resources to help it achieve this goal.

Education efforts at the annual meeting will play an essential role. Specifically, in the next 10 years we should have nationally known religion and health researchers as plenary speakers at least four times. In addition, every year for the next ten years we should have the following:

one or more pre-conference workshops that address the elements of research literacy, at least one pre-conference workshop for chaplains who wish to develop their own research projects, and workshops by chaplains presenting the results of their research. Further, regional and state chaplaincy meetings should contain workshops about research. After we have achieved our 10-year goal, research will no longer need to be such a priority for the national conference program, but it should always be an important component.

APC should also use its publications to support these research goals. Specifically, the APC newsletter should continue to have a regular research column. In addition, it should publish news of chaplains' participation in research projects and of their research publications. *Chaplaincy Today* should continue to publish research by chaplains and about chaplaincy, and the APC representative on the *Journal of Pastoral Care* board should support the publication of research that will be valuable to APC members.

The training of all new health care chaplains should help APC achieve and maintain these research goals. As the organization responsible for training the majority of board certified chaplains, the support of ACPE and its supervisors is essential to achieving this goal. Some CPE centers and supervisors already model and teach a research-informed approach to chaplaincy. Others will need to modify their curriculum or use adjunct faculty to help their students achieve these goals. During a one-year CPE residency, all students should learn to value research and become research literate. These two goals should also be added to the new ACPE Level II Outcomes. Some CPE programs have tried to teach their students how to do research during the residency year (Gibbons and Myler, 1978). Those programs should be encouraged to continue those efforts, but learning to do research should not become a goal for all one-year residency programs.

Changes in certification and continuing education policies will help reinforce the importance of these research goals for APC members and assist in monitoring our progress toward them. APC should require all candidates applying for certification as board certified chaplains to demonstrate that they value the importance of research for their ministry and are research literate. The candidate should present a short, written review of a well-conducted research article, summarizing its contents and describing their relevance for ministry. The APC policy about continuing education should be revised to specify that five of the required annual 50 continuing education hours (10%) should be research focused. This requirement could be fulfilled through courses, workshops, reading of research, or doing research.

The APC Research Committee should serve as a resource to the organization as it works to achieve and maintain these goals. It could provide names for speakers, workshop leaders and writers. It could foster communication among members who do research and help them network with research-focused individuals and organizations outside APC.

If APC made this 10-year commitment, I believe it could attract funding to reach these goals. This funding could support speakers and workshop leaders at state, regional, and national conferences. It could play a key role in helping some interested chaplains learn research skills by funding selected collaborative projects and providing scholarships for five or ten chaplains to complete a research degree such as a Masters in Public Health. The goals described here have been formulated in a measurable way and the funding could also be used to monitor our progress toward them.

CONCLUSION

As I stated at the beginning of this paper, the question is not whether to become a research-informed profession, but how to get there. I have described a ten-year strategy that enables the profession to become research-informed. These goals and steps are realistic. Making a commitment to become a research-informed profession in ten years is exciting and would win the support of various funding sources. I am excited to present this plan to my colleagues in APC and cognate groups for discussion, revision, and implementation. I am ready to lend my efforts to help it become a reality.

REFERENCES

Fitchett, G. (1999a). Screening for spiritual risk. *Chaplaincy Today*, 15(1): 2-12.
Fitchett, G. (1999b). Selected resources for screening for spiritual risk. *Chaplaincy Today* 15(1):13-26.
Fitchett, G., Meyer, P., & Burton, L. A. (2000). Spiritual care in the hospital: Who requests it? Who needs it? *Journal of Pastoral Care* 54(2): 173-186.

Gibbons, J., & Myler, D., Jr. (1978). Research as a curricular component in CPE. *Journal of Supervision and Training in Ministry* 1:36-45.

Iler, W., Obenshain, D., & Camac, M. (2001). The impact of daily visits from chaplains on patients with chronic obstructive pulmonary disease (COPD): A pilot study. *Chaplaincy Today*, 17(1), 5-11.

VandeCreek, L. & Lyon, M. (1997). *Ministry of Hospital Chaplains: Patient Satisfaction*. Binghamton, NY: The Haworth Pastoral Press.

Science and Ministry: Confusion and Reality

The Rev. George F. Handzo, MDiv, BCC

SUMMARY. The professional pastoral care community generates a great deal of heat but precious little light during its debate about the use of scientific process in the practice of ministry. This result is due in large part to confusion about the basic tasks and processes of science and its role in both organized religion and the current health care environment. Clergy have often not understood that science and faith are different enterprises, that science and art are overlapping processes, and that both science and ministry are means and not ends in themselves. In the current health care environment, the ability to use scientific processes and speak its language are not only essential to the survival of professional pastoral care but are necessary to promote the goals of pastoral care and enhance our ministry. *[Article copies available for a fee from The Haworth Document Delivery Service: 1-800-HAWORTH. E-mail address: <docdelivery@haworthpress.com> Website: <http://www.HaworthPress.com> © 2002 by The Haworth Press, Inc. All rights reserved.]*

KEYWORDS. Chaplaincy, pastoral care, ministry, science

The Rev. George F. Handzo is Director of Clinical Services, The HealthCare Chaplaincy, 307 East 70th Street, New York, NY 10022 (E-mail: ghandzo@heallthcarechaplaincy.org).

[Haworth co-indexing entry note]: "Science and Ministry: Confusion and Reality." Handzo, George F. Co-published simultaneously in *Journal of Health Care Chaplaincy* (The Haworth Pastoral Press, an imprint of The Haworth Press, Inc.) Vol. 12, No. 1/2, 2002, pp. 73-79; and: *Professional Chaplaincy and Clinical Pastoral Education Should Become More Scientific: Yes and No* (ed: Larry VandeCreek) The Haworth Pastoral Press, an imprint of The Haworth Press, Inc., 2003, pp. 73-79. Single or multiple copies of this article are available for a fee from The Haworth Document Delivery Service [1-800-HAWORTH, 9:00 a.m. - 5:00 p.m. (EST). E-mail address: docdelivery@haworthpress.com].

10.1300/J080v12n01_08

During the oral portion of my examination for ordination in the Lutheran church, one of the pastors on the committee noted my undergraduate degree in geology. With feeling bordering on accusation, he asked me how I could reconcile my training in science with my faith. It was clear that he believed that science and faith were incompatible and that I would have to forswear my scientific beliefs in order to become a pastor. I don' t remember my answer to the question, but, fortunately, the rest of the committee did not share this bias.

Although this pastor represents an extreme view, many religious people, especially religious professionals, do seem to harbor some belief that science and faith are antithetical. If you believe in the principles of one, you cannot with integrity believe in the principles of the other. To support this myth, we assume that no real scientist can be observantly religious. We try to ignore the fact that the current president of the American Psychiatric Association is an observant Seventh Day Adventist and that the current president of the American Society of Clinical Oncologists is an observant Jew. As with any stereotype, we treat these examples as aberrations that do not disprove the rule. If we can maintain that real scientists eschew religion, then we are safe in disavowing science.

The reality, as any good scientist will tell us, is that science and faith cannot be antithetical because they are two completely different enterprises. The basic distinction is that faith is a set of beliefs while science is a process. One could say that faith is knowledge, while science is a way to obtain knowledge. Faith is an end. Science is a means in the same way that Clinical Pastoral Education (CPE) is a means. One can talk about doing science just like one can talk about doing CPE. One would not talk about doing faith. An example of this problem occurs when scientific processes that demonstrate the helpfulness of religious belief and practice are also used to challenge (or demonstrate) the existence of God. Whether or not God exists is a matter of faith, not open to scientific inquiry. The effect of faith or religious practice on people's lives can be described by science irrespective of whether God exists or not. The same confusion occurs when skeptics view CPE as a challenge to religion or faith; in reality, it's a process for teaching people how to help others examine or affirm their faith.

Another confusion that seems a little harder to sort out–and one at the heart of this volume–is how the doing of science can fit into the doing of ministry. Here, we are comparing a process with a process. However, it seems the confusion often lies in our lack of clarity about means and ends. We often make the mistake of considering both science and ministry as ends when both are actually means to ends. Science is a means to acquire and use knowledge about the world around us and ministry is a means by which we help people come to faith and use that faith to guide their lives.

In reality, we all do science every day. It is part of the way we approach the world and communicate with one another. We are doing science when we think or talk about lengths or weights or anything where individual words have concrete equivalents. Science was and continues to be a major tool of the religious enterprise. We use science and the knowledge it produces to build houses of worship and to determine how best to communicate our faith to our children. Again, the important distinction is that science does not tell us what to teach, only how to teach it most effectively. More recently, the scientific process has helped us understand disease, especially psychological disease, in ways that have helped us counsel our congregants.

Those who oppose the increased role of science in chaplaincy seem to assume that the art of chaplaincy is incompatible with science. Some seem to define science as a purely rational process using evidence and conclusions based solely on numbers, whereas art is intuitive and based on individual judgment. In fact, what separates good scientists from others is their ability to intuit, to ask the right questions, to design elegant experiments that are works of art by any definition, and to see patterns and conclusions where others see chaos. Great scientists are those who have the ability to see when old models and paradigms no longer work and to create new models to fit the facts they see in front of them. If there were not an "art" to science, all scientists could be replaced with computers. Likewise, experienced chaplains are separated from neophytes by their ability to bring to any given patient the knowledge gained from hundreds of prior visits. When we use that knowledge, we are testing new data against existing models of behavior we have in our heads. We are doing science. By these definitions, there is no pure art or pure science. When we compare ministry and medicine, what we are really debating is the relative importance of "art" and "science" in the practice of each.

Now the discussion of one last confusion–the identification of science with the corporate influence on medicine. Certainly, the increased competition among health care institutions and the recent focus on cost have forced health care institutions to function much more like for-profit businesses than ever before. Processes like benchmarking that originated in the for-profit world are now common practice in not-for-profit health care. Outcome measures are increasingly prominent and drive medical decisions. Institutions are increasingly pressed to prove that they can, in fact, treat a given illness more effectively and cheaper than their competitors. Certainly, all of these processes are numbers driven. These numbers not only serve the goal of cutting cost but of demonstrating better outcomes than the competition. When Memorial Sloan-Kettering Cancer Center says in its ads that it provides "the best cancer care anywhere," it means that your chances of being cured are better if you are treated there than elsewhere, and it has lots of data to back up that claim. These data are not only the basis for marketing campaigns but for the crucial negotiations with third-party payers. Quality data of this kind will increasingly determine whether a given institution lives or dies. Health care institutions that think they can ignore this new reality or do not learn to deal with it expertly will be left behind and may cease to exist. They certainly did not choose this reality, but they have to learn to master it and even use it to their advantage. As a health care administrator I know likes to say, "He who has the best data wins."

This emphasis on efficiency and outcomes, however, is as irritating to the scientists as it is to those in ministry. The push for immediate results makes it very difficult to justify the "basic sciences" because they do not produce immediate patient benefits. Likewise, the costly training of new practitioners does not produce patient benefits commensurate with its expense. The rise of the corporate model in medicine, while it makes heavy use of scientific processes, cannot be blamed on science or scientists. How and why we are in this place in American health care is a socio-political question far beyond the scope of this paper. Hardly anyone in health care likes this reality. However, the prospering individuals and institutions have not only acknowledged it but have learned to use it to their advantage.

Since the health care culture increasingly depends on number-driven outcome measures, chaplains need to decide how, as pastoral care professionals, they are going to respond. In formulating that response, they need to remember that the goals of ministry in health care are not necessarily the same as those in congregational ministry where preaching and teaching the Word of God is an end in itself. Whether that preaching and teaching has an effect on any individual is not necessarily relevant. In the health care setting, the goal, or end, can be formulated in various ways. Chaplain Yes and Chaplain No express one formulation at the beginning of this volume: "to represent the love of the Transcendent during illness, despair, and death." Another that I have used is "assist those who are suffering to maximize their religious and spiritual resources in the service of coping." However we formulate this goal, it necessitates being present with those who suffer in ways that promote their spiritual well being. Most formulations of this goal imply or state that what we do helps people who are suffering. In other words, our ministry has a positive outcome. The goal also includes promoting respect for individuals. Any response we make in this current environment must be measured against this goal. If the response does not promote this end, it must be rejected. We must look for the response that most promotes this goal.

The first possible response involves non-cooperation with this new culture. We simply go about business as always. Those who oppose the use of science in chaplaincy implicitly advocate this approach. Given this response, professional chaplaincy may continue to exist in institutions with small pastoral care budgets or where religious communities are significantly involved. Even in those settings, however, institutional administrators have often already figured out that regulations do not require professional chaplains. The Joint Commission on the Accreditation of Health Care Organizations will be perfectly happy with an effective network of on-call community clergy that costs the institution little or nothing.

To opt out of the corporate culture leaves the future of professional pastoral care in the hands of others. In some cases, local religious communities will rally to the chaplain's defense and carry the day. In many cases, seeing no evidence (i.e., data), professional pastoral care will be eliminated. Chaplains can then stand outside the hospital walls, feeling virtuous that they have not sold out, and rail against the evils of the corporate culture. The problem is that the patients, families and staff we previously served and who still need us will continue to be inside the walls and will continue to suffer without the benefit of our ministry. In the service of being pure and prophetic, we will have abdicated our calling and abandoned those who need us. The goal of ministry will not be served. We may say it is not our fault, but, in fact, the choice will have been ours.

Another strategy involves changing the corporate culture or at least modifying it in ways that are more to our liking. This is a worthy goal and one we should undertake. However, in the pursuit of this goal, we must focus on practices and policies that truly impede the delivery of pastoral care rather than simply trying to make life easier for us. By example, the HIPPA regulations that were expected become fully effective during 2002 may very well restrict the chaplain's ability to go room to room, visiting patients who have not asked to be visited. Professional chaplaincy will then depend completely on the referrals of others. This change will necessitate a fundamental shift in the delivery of pastoral care. While chaplains will find a great deal of legitimate fault with these regulations, they are based on the patient's right to privacy and confidentiality–rights we have long championed. Any challenge to these regulations must be done carefully and clearly from the patient's perspective lest the challenge appear self serving and hypocritical. It can easily appear that we are for the patient's right to be protected from uninvited visits only until it infringes on our professional practice.

In any case, changing individual regulations or the culture of health care, while a worthy goal, cannot likely be a short-term goal for the individual practitioner–although pastoral care organizations certainly need make it part of their long-term agenda in cooperation with other professional groups. However, if this is our only response, many chaplaincy positions will be lost while we pursue it, again resulting in the goal not being served.

If we are clear about our goal and dedicated to it, we should be willing to use reasonable and ethical means to achieve and maximize it. The use of scientific process does not necessarily change the goal of pastoral care. Scientific methodology is only a means, and one we in organized religion continue to use to our advantage to achieve our ends in other settings. As long as we keep the goal of our ministry firmly in mind, science will not corrupt or co-opt our ministry.

On the contrary, scientific language is the universally understood means of communication in our culture. To pass up the scientific process as a way to communicate what we are about or even as a way to maximize the effectiveness of what we do passes up a major tool at our disposal for achieving the goals of our ministry. To enter the world of health care and not be able to speak in the language of science is like undertaking missionary work in a foreign country and speaking only English. There will be those who understand us, but our work will largely be ineffective because of the language barrier.

If we believe that our ministry helps people, we should certainly want it to help as many people as possible. The proponents of many so called "alternative therapies" like meditation and acupuncture are successfully using this new emphasis on outcomes in medicine to demonstrate that their therapies actually help people and are cost effective. As noted above, our professed goal in health care ministry at least implies that what we do helps reduce suffering. If we really want to be accepted as a full part of a treatment team as we have long proclaimed, we now have an opportunity to demonstrate that we should be fully integrated.

Of course, dangers exist. As a profession, we have not been terribly accountable for what we do in the health care setting. We have functioned on the fringe of our religious organizations and the health care institutions have often accepted us "on faith." Additionally, becoming more scientific may reveal that some of our practices do not help people. We may need to abandon or revise some of our cherished practices. Again, the goal will not change, but our means may need to be altered.

In sum, science is not a challenge to faith nor is it our enemy. The corporate emphasis on outcomes is not our enemy. Both science and outcome measures are processes that are neither good nor evil in themselves. They are means that become good or evil depending on the use to which we put them. We are presented now with a choice. We can divert our energies from helping those who are suffering to play the victim and decry the evil forces that surround us. Alternatively, we can learn how to use these processes to our advantage, and, more importantly, to the advantage of those who are suffering and need the spiritual care that we provide.

Siblings or Foes:
What Now in Spiritual Care Research?

Gordon J. Hilsman, DMin, BCC

SUMMARY. This article uses a sibling metaphor to outline the relation-ship between science and spirituality. This metaphor forms the backdrop for exploring several directions in spiritual care research. It argues that science and functional spirituality were born as siblings and need to dance now without either estrangement or incest, intent on measuring the material effects of excellent pastoral care. *[Article copies available for a fee from The Haworth Document Delivery Service: 1-800-HAWORTH. E-mail address: <docdelivery@haworthpress.com> Website: <http://www.HaworthPress.com> © 2002 by The Haworth Press, Inc. All rights reserved.]*

KEYWORDS. Spiritual care, spirituality, chaplaincy, research

Many professional chaplains are currently perched on the fence about measurement in spiritual care. Literally hundreds of studies con-ducted in the past fifteen years confirm what has been known anecdotally for centuries: sensitive and savvy pastoral care adds value to the human person and resilience to people in crisis.[1] Ought this research movement

Gordon J. Hilsman is Manager of Clinical Pastoral Education in the Spiritual Care Team, Franciscan Health System, Tacoma, WA (E-mail: gordonhilsman@chiwest.com).

[Haworth co-indexing entry note]: "Siblings or Foes: What Now in Spiritual Care Research?" Hilsman, Gordon J. Co-published simultaneously in *Journal of Health Care Chaplaincy* (The Haworth Pastoral Press, an imprint of The Haworth Press, Inc.) Vol. 12, No. 1/2, 2002, pp. 81-89; and: *Professional Chaplaincy and Clinical Pastoral Education Should Become More Scientific: Yes and No* (ed: Larry VandeCreek) The Haworth Pastoral Press, an imprint of The Haworth Press, Inc., 2003, pp. 81-89. Single or multiple copies of this article are available for a fee from The Haworth Document Delivery Service [1-800-HAWORTH, 9:00 a.m. - 5:00 p.m. (EST). E-mail address: docdelivery@haworthpress.com].

now be stopped in order to protect our uniqueness or enhanced to further establish our effectiveness? Is science our friend or our foe? A brief historical context may contribute perspective concerning which option offers the more promise.

A CONJECTURED HISTORICAL CONTEXT

Science and spirituality, distinct as they are, emerged together and flourished in different ages. They both grew out of the same human experience, namely facing the ambiguity of unfathomable mystery. When the first individual, however primitive, began to record the regularity of the moon's movements, s/he began to add scientific analyses to already established spiritual responses to that obvious orb's enchanting aura. The measurement and usefulness of science became brother to the shared awe of aboriginal spirituality.

Science and religion are indeed like feisty siblings, a brother and a sister who emerged from the same pristine origins, yet see each other as rivals and perceive the world as differently as stereotypical man and woman. They "scuffled" over visionaries like Galilei Galileo and Charles Darwin, and came closest to enmeshment during the decades when alchemy and magic stubbornly attempted to create gold. For the most part, however, they stayed individuated, respecting their differences and dancing occasionally, while avoiding estrangement on the one hand and incest on the other.

Spirituality was probably the first-born, and is more "of the heart." Mysterious natural phenomena, such as the moon, the sun, the stars, the wind, the luck of the hunt and the fury of the mountain storm, no doubt prompted not only awe but also efforts to honor and influence their unknown powers. The more internal experiences, such as illness, disabling wounds, fertility/infertility, arthritic pain, sexual rhythms and death, were probably no less inscrutable and fascinating. These unpredictable, mysterious forces compelled attention.

Innumerable methods that sought to appreciate and influence these phenomena eventually clustered together into beliefs, practices, myths, stories, and art that constituted primitive religions. Ways of enjoying life while coping with the dangerous beauty of the natural, relational and inner worlds constitute what we call spiritual practice.

Spirituality as functional, i.e., as valued for what it effects in the human experience, constituted an array of beliefs, practices, habits and values that an individual employs to help her/him cope with and enjoy the aspects of life s/he could not control. Spiritual coping and enjoyment eventually included some focus on the inscrutable quality of human relationships with self and others, as well as with *The Beyond.* Such terms as love, care, worship, awe, sin, reconciliation, support, hope, faith, prayer, spirit and soul became a "Babel" of multi-meaning terms by which to converse about what was inherently beyond comprehension. As these various methods were shared, taught, articulated, perpetuated, systematized and utilized in a communal context, they could (in admittedly Christian terminology) be said to constitute faith communities or churches.[2]

Science, on the other hand, focused on the world of material reality, using the budding cognitive capacities of evolving humans to gain some power, to do things better, and to improve the species. More focused on "effective doing" than "appreciative enjoying," science worked with technology, its brother that specialized in the use of science to improve living. They flourished together in fire cooking, home building, agriculture and weaponry. Various societies notably advanced the state of science and technology, notably the ancient Chinese, the Egyptians, the Aztecs, the Enlightened Europeans and more recently the North Americans.

As science and technology progressed (the boys got bigger than their sister!), they overshadowed the inherently mysterious nature of the universe. Science took a piece of reality and attempted to move it from unfathomable mystery to useful technology via a disciplined process of hypothesis, experiment, measurement, theorizing and confirmation through further experimentation and re-measurement. A few hundred years ago for example, what glowed in the dark clearly fit into the religion-spiritual arena, until it was "explained" by the science of electromagnetic waves.

Science tends to view as "real" and place value only on what is "proven." It produces a seductive and misleading impression of certitude. Thus, human emotion has little place in science, except as science is able to contribute to comfort, security and health. Even the "soft science" of psychology classically has not included such words as "love" and "forgiveness" in its research efforts, presumably due to their elusive "spiritual" nature. Science only deals with what it can measure, has measured or can conceive of how to measure (although scientists too must go home at night compelled to awe at the sight of the un-measurable smiles and giggles of their sons and daughters).

The universe, however, remains inherently mysterious, despite several hundred years of measurement. Mystery could be defined as a reality so complex that it can never be comprehended, though it tends to further unfold the more deeply one enters into it. Romantic love, human care, the processes of dying and nurturing of children are obvious examples. But upon close examination, all aspects of life are a mystery. Religion and science are two ways of addressing mysteries' unsettling unpredictability. One could say that health care chaplains are evolving religion-spiritual practitioners functioning in a scientific/technological world. These siblings are attempting to dance anew within attempts to measure spiritual care outcomes.

THE CHAPLAINCY DILEMMA

Professional chaplaincy is a product of both religion and the softer sciences, born in this country in a 1920s mission of melding Christian traditions and Freudian-energized behavioral sciences.[3] Chaplaincy, as a religious means to support people at times of personal crisis and loss, had already existed in the Roman Catholic tradition for centuries. That "denominational Chaplaincy" used traditionally developed religious practices such as prayer, rituals, sacred words and sacraments to assist people's coping with "bad things happening."

"Professional Chaplaincy" however, was born of compassion in the midst of diversity in religious practice and attitude, a response to a perceived call to care spiritually for people in the public institutions of a pluralistic society. From that perspective it became pragmatically ineffective to operate entirely from one's own religious tradition. An entire new field of care came into existence, a field that sought to combine the best of religious traditions and the newly developing behavioral sciences. It focused on the question of "What is best personally for this individual in this painful situation?" The new professional chaplaincy was person-centered rather than proceeding from assumptions of "absolute truth," or the favorite theological systems of religious practitioners.

While it developed initially in psychiatric settings, the fledgling professional chaplaincy movement spread to general hospitals where its mission was more directed at assisting people with what might today be called "unwanted outcomes" such as dying and the threat of disability and death. It mixed day to day with the medical model of care, which was heavily absorbed in artistically applying science and technology to improving and prolonging life. To oversimplify, when medicine no longer helped, chaplaincy cared. Since professional chaplaincy developed primarily in the U.S., the influence of the American philosophy of Pragmatism was influential. Founded by John Dewey and briefly summarized as "whatever works best is best," it contributed to the already established American "can do" ethos and the New World explosion of technology to improve human life with comfort and convenience. The Alcoholics Anonymous movement, born in New York and Akron in the 1930s, and enormously effective in its sphere of influence, features major pragmatic elements, as do many of the service professions spawned from nursing during the twentieth century. Orthopedic patients, for example, walked sooner with physical therapy, which can be "proven" through research as well as anecdotally observed.

A revival of Empiricism, or the emphasis on valuing what can be measured, now combined with pragmatism to fuel the current impetus for research in spiritual care. We are urged to "prove" that the caring of professional chaplaincy works; it improves people's lives. Science is now chiding its sister religion to bend to scientific methodology, much as religion leaned on science to conform to its "truth" regarding astronomy in the seventeenth century and evolution in the nineteenth century.

The "wellness" or "wholism" themes in health care constitutes a more recent contribution to the current thrust to produce research in spiritual care. "Being well" is more than "being healthy by medical observation," as heart attack victims without previous symptoms can testify. Wellness and risk factors can partially be observed where no symptoms are yet seen. Entire health systems began to adopt "community wellness" missions, goals and initiatives.[4]

This shift in health care mission challenged chaplaincy. Even though traditionally focused on helping people deal with the unwanted aspects of life, chaplaincy is now compelled into the current thrusts of "wellness," "improving the health of communities" and "outcomes research." We are actually being invited to transform, or perhaps catalyze, the evolution of our profession from our roots in spiritual assistance to painful situations, to enhancing people's lives through augmenting their perspective on health with those of spiritual traditions and care–all this, while measuring how well we do it and how much it helps.

CONFRONTING THE "BOGGLE FACTOR"

But science and religion tend to stay stubbornly individuated from one another. Internist author Larry Dossey[5] coined the term "boggle factor," referring to the intangible limit of what people will let themselves believe regarding research on spirituality. No matter how clearly spirituality is measured, people accustomed to the assurance of scientific measurement will go only so far in believing measurements of the spiritual. The multitude of studies on spiritual care effects done in the 1980s and 1990s were conducted from the diverse perspectives of physicians,[6] chaplains,[7] psychologists[8] and large healthcare systems[9] interested in the integration of spirituality into the scientific/technological healthcare world. But readers will go only so far in believing that spiritual experience actually contributes to physical healing, or even that its effects on personal healing are significant. Something "boggles our minds" when proof of spiritual power is asserted too clearly or solidly.

Yet this research work has not gone in vain. It has helped focus pastoral staffs, encouraged and contributed direction to their continuing education efforts. It has motivated some managers and administrators to follow their own intuitive sense that supporting spiritual care integration into healthcare systems makes good sense. And it has given focus and substance to spiritual care directors as they have approached administrative leaders for support.

But the endeavor of measuring the material results of spiritual caring will never prove its healing efficacy to the satisfaction of scientific practitioners. Like all aspects of scientific study, it is endless. Progress is made slowly and continuously, not definitively and once-and-for-all. Such efforts need to continue but ought not overshadow the care itself. We must overcome the fear that the stronger younger brother will rape the more vulnerable older sister. They can dance.

DANCING WITHIN BOUNDARIES

As the siblings dance in new ways regarding spiritual care in scientific/technological arenas, there are some steps to be respected. They need the structure of a waltz, jig or tango more than the "move however you like" modern day cavorting. In other words, while research continues in the area of the spiritual care effects on persons, four guidelines for our professional direction may be helpful. They are: (1) carefully design and collaborate on our studies to create excellent research; (2) continually enhance the quality of our care itself to create excellent care; (3) focus on integration of what has already been studied; and (4) rigorously respect our limitations.

1. Carefully decide what to study. Let us focus our study. Science itself takes small bites at a time, pecking away at what is measurable. Neither will it prove spiritual care's efficacy "once and for all." Science has made huge progress in the past 500 years, but that progress is minuscule *vis a vis* the mysteries that make up the universe. Our attitude needs to be one of evolutionary pace, careful selection of hypotheses and excellence of research project, to keep our effect and our value constantly visible.

Psychologist Mary van de Groot, in *Narrating Psychology,*[10] once outlined how the field of psychology was formed by what it decided to study and what it chose not to address. We too will be influenced as a profession by what we choose to examine and what is essentially "taboo." How will we decide what studies are most beneficial to the people for whom we care?

Collaboration of leaders in professional chaplaincy organizations, along with those gifted in measurement of spiritual care parameters, could well focus half of our studies with both imagination and perspicacious discernment of optimal usefulness. The other half of studies need to be left to whatever individuals' own intuition inspires them to study. At this point in history, evolution moves ahead both by individual inspiration and astute communal collaboration. And we need to build on previous studies, rather than "reinventing the wheel" that may have been studied previously.

Research is not for everyone. Quality counts amid professional researchers who will no doubt critique any significant studies of spiritual care. If you must do research, seek continuing education and regular consultation. It is an endeavor that is as profoundly different from chaplaincy as science is from religion. Like pastoral care it must be learned through experience and feedback.

2. Stubbornly and creatively focus on quality of care. Our studies need to continually prompt us to improve the excellence of our spiritual care. Stubbornly focusing on the quality of our care is essential, since only excellence of care is worth measuring. Research can easily distract us from what is effectively pastoral, to what is politically attractive. The benefits of consultation with one another need to be a persistent characteristic of our ongoing practice, not just the nature of our formative education.

3. Integrate what has already been proven. The current most urgent call and challenge of chaplaincy and Clinical Pastoral Education is not measurement, but integration. Thomas Moore in *Soul Care*[11] has suggested that we have known for a long time that mind and body are connected in intricate ways, but that we will continue to make little progress on integrating them in health care until we focus more on the soul. How will we maximize the effects of our research in the politics and culture of healthcare settings? Integration is a complex process in any single human life. How far can health care systems integrate without some focus on the personal integration of practitioners, managers and administrators alike? Taboos aside, as the person with the least capacity for intimacy sets the relational level of closeness, so the people with the most "siloed" or "compartmentalized" patterns of working together, act as bottlenecks in the integration of body, mind and spirit in care settings and corporations. Let us clarify the role of chaplaincy in the ongoing integration of spiritual perspectives into healthcare structures.

One thrust of integration will include seeking leadership and funding from our corporate systems. They may eventually embrace the idea of spiritual care research and see its value. Studies done by untrained researches with philosophical minds on little or no funding for design, consultation and costs, will likely be of meager benefit.

4. Deeply respect our limitations. Chaplaincy has always been an endeavor that assists people in the meeting of limitations, and here we need to respect our own limitations regarding measurement. We can't make researchers out of all chaplains. Facility for research design, using scientific frameworks, is not evenly distributed among us. Unless you have both an interest and a charism for disciplined study, leave the research to the experts. Many chaplains best refuse to become overly pre-occupied with research. No more than five percent of a chaplain's efforts ought to be spent in measuring anything. About one percent is probably the maximum for most of us.

CONCLUSION

Chaplains who see science and spirituality as having similar pristine roots, followed by persistent intertwining and skirmishing throughout human history, are likely now to be confident that measurement in spiritual care need not destroy the profession. Nor will it either elevate it to certitude or devalue it to "just another behavioral science." Both the cognitive scientific view and the heartfelt spiritual one are inherent perspectives of the human species, and they are both here to stay, compelled to respect one another as viable engagements of the inherently mysterious world. What comes of our research on outcomes of spiritual care needs to help guide us in being "in the world but not of it," rather than frighten us with fears of being obliterated on the one hand or engulfed on the other. Our best approach is to foster quality research in our field, collaborate on what we consider to be the best research directions in any given era, use our imaginations to employ the research results into our continually developing and refining of care, and invest constantly in the process of integrating spiritual perspectives into all of health care.

NOTES

1. Psychologist Kenneth I. Pargament has spent years studying and teaching about the resilience religious practice and belief contribute to a person's psychological makeup and coping. See for example, Kenneth I. Pargament, *The Psychology of Religion and Coping: Theory, Research, Practice* (The Guilford Press: New York, 1997) and Dale A. Mathews, MD, *The Faith Factor: Proof of the Healing Power of Prayer* (Viking Penquin, 1998).

2. Ted Fortier, PhD, advises me that suggesting that these changes in spiritual and religious practice actually evolved, or *improved* over time, is anthropologically questionable. From the anthropological point of view, who is to say they are actually better now than they were in what I am calling their earlier forms? (Tedf@Seattleu.edu).

3. Charles E. Hall, *Head and Heart: The Story of the Clinical Pastoral Education Movement*, (Decatur GA, Journal of Pastoral Care, 1992).

4. For example, the stated mission of Catholic Health Initiatives, the nation's largest Catholic health system formed in 1995, states in part, "Fidelity to the Gospel urges us to emphasize human dignity and social justice as we move towards healthier communities."

5. Dossey has used this term in public addresses in at least two places, at the Providence Health System in Seattle in 1995 and at the ACPE/AAPC joint national annual conference in Albuquerque in 1999.

6. Research leaders among physicians have been some of the most credible to healthcare practitioners. Dossey himself cites studies of how heart patients heal faster and bacteria grow better under the influence of prayer, given that the person praying actually can generate feelings of love for the patient or the bacteria. David B. Larson at the National Institutes of Health and Dale E. Mathews at Georgetown are, like Dossey, physicians who value the "faith factor" in healing and are bent on studying its power to contribute to personal healing. All of these augment the bold and well known earliest studies with orthopedic patients at the VA Medical Center in West Roxbury, MA published by physician Elizabeth McSherry in 1986, clearly documenting the efficacy of pastoral intervention ("*Pastoral Care Departments: More Necessary in the DRG Era,*" *Heath Care Management Review*, (Win) 1986, Vol. 11, No. 1, pp. 47-59).

7. Larry VandeCreek and George Fitchette, Chaplains and CPE Supervisors, have authored and co-authored a wide variety of similar studies from the pastoral perspective.

8 Op. cit., Pargament.

9. Bartholomew Rodrigues et al., *Spiritual Needs & Chaplaincy Services: A National Empirical Study on Chaplaincy Encounters in Health Care Settings*, was commissioned and coordinated by The Providence Health System on the west coast in early 2000 (Providence Health System: 2000).

10. Mary Vander Groot, *Narrating Psychology: Or, How Psychology Gets Made,* (Wyndham Hall Press, 1987).

11. Thomas Moore, *Care of the Soul* (Harper Collins, 1992), p. xv and Chapter 8, "*The Body's Poetics of Illness,*" pp. 155-176.

Research or Perish?

Margot Hover, DMin

SUMMARY. The opportunity for sound pastoral care research is not served by the "all or nothing" approach. Professional chaplains whose training includes a thorough orientation to the research process are in a position to speak to the world of science about realities that are beyond physical research, and to the world of theology about realities that should be examined. Cloning, embryonic experimentation, and drug trials in Third World populations are among the areas without the voices of pastoral theologians. Closer to daily practice, research is an invaluable tool in helping chaplains improve their ministry. *[Article copies available for a fee from The Haworth Document Delivery Service: 1-800-HAWORTH. E-mail address: <docdelivery@haworthpress.com> Website: <http://www.HaworthPress.com> © 2002 by The Haworth Press, Inc. All rights reserved.]*

KEYWORDS. Chaplaincy, clinical pastoral education, research, pastoral care

Several years ago, I was part of an interdisciplinary group that spent six months in discussions on prayer, spirituality and religiosity as it related to physical health. All of us agreed that much of the research to

Margot Hover is Clinical Pastoral Educator, Barnes Jewish Hospital, St. Louis, MO 63111 (E-mail: hoverm@mskmail.mskcc.org).

[Haworth co-indexing entry note]: "Research or Perish?" Hover, Margot. Co-published simultaneously in *Journal of Health Care Chaplaincy* (The Haworth Pastoral Press, an imprint of The Haworth Press, Inc.) Vol. 12, No. 1/2, 2002, pp. 91-97; and: *Professional Chaplaincy and Clinical Pastoral Education Should Become More Scientific: Yes and No* (ed: Larry VandeCreek) The Haworth Pastoral Press, an imprint of The Haworth Press, Inc., 2003, pp. 91-97. Single or multiple copies of this article are available for a fee from The Haworth Document Delivery Service [1-800-HAWORTH, 9:00 a.m. - 5:00 p.m. (EST). E-mail address: docdelivery@haworthpress.com].

10.1300/J080v12n01_10

that point was inadequate. Week after week, we debated issues, definitions and conclusions from the standpoint of our various disciplines–ethics, philosophy, medicine, psychology, and pastoral care. Responses to a publication by the group were forwarded to us for response. I was somewhat taken aback by the vehemence of the attacks that I received as the chaplain ("You have sold your soul to the devil!"), particularly from some of the clergy.

However, I wasn't surprised either by the volume of responses or by the range of opinions. Religion and health is a current "hot issue." What I did find surprising were the assumptions about what chaplains do. By and large, they were consistent with the stereotypes held by many of our peers in the other healthcare professions. If physicians, nurses and technicians have had a good experience with church or clergy, they assume that we're sensitive and intuitive and generally helpful. In the words of a fellow committee member years ago, "What harm can a chaplain do with a little questionnaire?" What harm can a chaplain do with a little pastoral visit? And the converse is true as well: If other staff's personal and/or professional relationships with church or clergy have been painful, they put us in the "irrelevant" or "harmful" box. But both groups with embarrassing frequency assumed that chaplains' preparation for their work consisted solely of some call from the Divine; they were surprised to learn that specialized education was part of that preparation. I must note here that in terms of my own theology, neither excludes the other. My ministry proceeds from my gifts and love for the work, and the endorsement of my skill by my denomination and other certifying bodies; both constitute my "Call."

I found another surprising facet of the experience. Each time the chaplains pushed for space to define our position or support our arguments, we were labeled "defensive" and "territorial." That would never be said of a neurosurgeon or clinical nurse specialist–or social worker. But that argument effectively silenced our voices on some crucial points that pertain specifically to our discipline.

If only we could let matters ride along as they have thus far; some healthcare institutions have chaplains; some don't, and that's fine. However, the ante goes up each time the American healthcare system faces an economic crunch. Dollars and positions become scarce, and each discipline scrambles for the "Next New Thing" that will secure their place at the table as well as in the institution's budget. We remember the New Things of past and more recent decades. Cancer patients in the 80s were certain that guided imagery was the key to the effectiveness of their chemotherapy, and so they meditated faithfully on PacMen gobbling up their cancer cells each time they received a treatment. And now, it appears that spirituality is the New Thing of this era. But look at the rosters of speakers at forums, workshops and seminars on spirituality, medicine and healthcare. Where are the chaplains? Many of the best selling authors in the area of spirituality and health profess strong personal faith but no systematic theological training. How many of the titles concerning spirituality and health are contributed by religious professionals in the field?

So this is the climate. And the question posed to us is this: Should clinical pastoral education and professional chaplaincy become more scientific in response to health care reform? At the risk of seeming to have no opinion, I advocate strongly for all three: Yes! No! It depends!

First, it is important here to define terms. Scientific investigation is, at bottom, the process of ordering our observations (Southard, 1976). The process education model at the heart of Clinical Pastoral Education (CPE) consists of a series of intervention studies in which students visit patients or participate in peer groups. They then reflect on that experience through the lens of their individualized learning contract, the pastoral work presentation or verbatim outline, and the Standards and Outcomes of the various levels of CPE. Their subsequent pastoral practice is illuminated and informed by the feedback they receive and by their reflection on that process, using the traditional model of our discipline–action, reflection, action. In that sense, CPE has always revolved around the systematic ordering of student and supervisor observations. It is already scientific, and was so long before the most recent healthcare reform.

I suspect, however, that "more scientific" in the current dialogue unfortunately means prayer studies of the type done in by Randolph Byrd (1988). Research in pastoral care, spirituality and religiosity is much broader, more useful and ethically and theologically more defensible than that approach. For example, one of the most valuable outcomes of any research project is the sharpening of definitions that occurs in the preliminary stages of setting up a study. If the initial question is "How do patients feel about chaplains?"–a satisfaction survey–one immediately begins to see that each term must be narrowed over and over. In-patients or outpatients? Those who have been visited by a chaplain during that hospitalization or those who haven't? Long term or same-day surgery patients? Those who regularly attend worship or those unaffiliated with a particular congregation or parish? Those with strong networks of social support or those who are isolated for one reason or another?

And then the "chaplain" term of the research question: did the chaplain supply the religious services patients wished and expected? Was the chaplain experienced or a student? Where was the visit done–immediately pre-surgery, pre-admission, telephone call post admission, emergency room, in the company of the physician delivering news, following a death to address the issue of organ donation? How long was the visit, and were there follow-up visits? As we wonder about those questions simply in refining the initial one, we begin to look at our practice more carefully and strategically. For some time now, chaplains have used research to plan coverage, to see when visits to what patients will be most helpful (Fitchett et al., 2000).

So one contribution of research in our discipline is that it improves and sharpens our effectiveness as pastoral care givers. The second value of research is that it helps us to communicate what we do to our co-workers in other disciplines. The purpose of such communication is not "to sell ourselves," but to clarify our role in partnership with the rest of the healthcare team so that we can be appropriately and effectively used in the care of patients. It is clear that the convener of our discussion group thought that we as religious professionals had something to contribute to the dialogue; he wasn't at all clear about what that might be. Several months later, he read something I wrote on the assessment of spiritual injury, in which I spoke specifically in terms that are the vocabulary of spiritual diagnosis in our hospital. "I didn't know you did all that!" he exclaimed. That indicated to me that his stereotypes of chaplains were so imbedded that I had to use clinical terminology parallel in sophistication to his in order to break through them. I had nothing to gain by "selling myself" in his setting, but I did need to convince him that the issue he undertook to address was beyond the expertise of his field alone; he needed us. The traditional language of CPE and pastoral care–"walking with" patients, "standing with" them, and "feeling their pain" did not communicate that.

I am convinced that professional chaplains must be able to understand and to speak the language appropriate to their setting if they are to be taken seriously there. For example, in the early years of Institutional Review Boards and Human Subjects Committees, a chaplain might be included, and expected to begin meetings with a prayer. Period! Later, it was assumed that the chaplain or local clergy representative served as the watchdog on ethical issues. By now, in many institutions where research is done, it is assumed that chaplain IRB members understand the research process, and can contribute to the dialogue around protocols in important, even crucial ways. Further–and this on an institution-by-institution basis only–chaplains submit their own protocols, and so demonstrate to their peers in other disciplines that they have mastered a skill that is already part of every other health profession.

I find the suggestion that we as chaplains have "sold out" by learning and doing research in our field ludicrous and demeaning. We wouldn't accuse a chaplain who can recognize the signs of clinical depression of "selling out" to the field of psychology or psychiatry. On the contrary, we should assume that a professional chaplain should be able to recognize depression, for instance, in order to make an appropriate referral. Following the same argument, it seems to me that every professional chaplain should at least be able to read research with discrimination, and should be able to set up and implement simple research projects that would illuminate and enrich her practice as a chaplain. We expect a CPE curriculum to include didactics on group formation and dynamics, and we don't see that as "selling out" to the field of psychology. It's not clear to me what the chaplain researcher has sold out *to*.

Having said all that, now to the argument by Chaplain No found in the opening pages of this volume–or at least in that direction. In the world of health care, only the chaplain researcher stands between the physical sciences and spirituality, able to speak to both. The chaplain researcher reminds physical scientists that some issues cannot be researched, and s/he reminds the pastoral theologian that some issues can and should be researched. A case in point: Studies on non-local intercessory prayer are critiqued on a number of procedural points. For example, how was it insured that the "No prayer" participants were not actually prayed for during the study? Were the outcome measures appropriate to the research question? How was the intervention–prayer–defined and limited? Chaplains should be able to raise those questions with authority, since we are the specialists in religious practice and spirituality.

Further, it is the place of pastoral theologians–chaplains–to critique the basic assumptions on which these studies are based–that the purpose of prayer is functional, and that prayer "works" in the same as medications. It is undeniable that human beings tend to look at religious ritual in terms of what it will persuade God to do, particularly about those situations where they feel powerless. Nevertheless, the pastoral theologian reminds the scientist that many of the world religions regard prayer as primarily a relationship with the Divine; to value prayer primarily for what it accomplishes for us trivializes spirituality.

So I believe that the voice of professional chaplains should be heard in the realm of clinical research for the sake of the integrity, quality and direction of research in pastoral care and spirituality, not merely to buy ourselves a guaranteed piece of the healthcare economic pie. This obviously means that research must be included in the CPE curriculum, particularly for students intending a career in chaplaincy. Among the Objectives for accredited ACPE programs (2001) is "the ability to make effective use of . . . the behavioral sciences in pastoral ministry to persons and groups." The outcomes for Level One focus on self-awareness, basic pastoral skills, and processes for ongoing professional development and review. The Outcomes for Level II focus more on specific clinical skills.

While my previous arguments emphasize the role of research as pastoral theologians speak to their peers in other disciplines, these standards and outcomes focus on the role of research in the religious professional's organization and assessment of her own work. VandeCreek and colleagues (1994) lift up a cardinal principle in their rationale for the doing and teaching of research in our field: "The world and human experience are more complicated than they appear." Of course, we knew that. But we do tend to look for insight and help with the "more complicated" in the theological and psychological–if we look at all. When I take an honest look at how I do pastoral care and supervision, an amazing proportion of my practice is "because I learned it that way," or "because I've always done it that way." And while I've continued to do many things "that way" because they seem effective, what would I stand to lose if I looked at them through the lens of research? For example, what might I gain if I kept track of former students who got–and kept–jobs in the field of pastoral care? What would I learn if I compared the satisfaction of patients who received an informational visit from a hospital volunteer with patients who receive a spiritual assessment from a chaplain?–or a nurse?–or a clerk in Pre-admission Testing? Would my priorities and practice change if I counted referrals and noticed an increase around the time I began attending unit Multidisciplinary Rounds or began to write notes in the charts of patients?

These represent a random sample of practice issues about which chaplains should be curious about–regardless of how busy they are each day. Business is an indisputable fact but poor excuse for neglecting the critical reading of research in our field and actually doing at least simple quality assurance studies of "the way we do things."

"Tell me where is fancy bred;/In the heart or in the head?/How begot, how nourished? Reply, reply," sings Shakespeare's troubadour in *Merchant of Venice* (no date). It's unfortunate that the various voices in the discussion of the appropriateness, place, and "goodness of fit" between research, pastoral theology and spiritual care have become so polarized.

Spirituality is "bred" by the union between heart and head. The best-selling novelist Mark Salzman nibbles around the edges of the issue of ultimate meaning versus rationality in his earlier novels, but he seems to take the question more seriously in his most recent novel, *Lying Awake* (2000). Sister John of the Cross, a middle-aged Carmelite nun, finds her years of spiritual dryness recently interrupted by waking dreams of rapturous religious ecstasy. Eventually, these "spells" are diagnosed as a non-malignant temporal lobe tumor. The story turns on her dilemma; if the tumor is removed, will her visions cease and her desert return? Her surgeon is quite blithe about her recovery, not understanding at all the implications of the surgery for her spirituality–in her heart and soul. Ultimately, Sister John finds affirmation and solace in her decision by remembering her "very first prayer at Carmel, when Mother Mary Joseph told her to kneel before the altar and make her wishes known to God. Please, God, let me know you. If God's mystery only deepens as we learn about him, she thought, then maybe he's been answering my prayer after all" (p. 179). As chaplains, we can and should bear articulate witness to both the mystery and the learning.

REFERENCES

Association for Clinical Pastoral Education. (2001). The Standards of The Association for Clinical Pastoral Education. Decatur, GA: Association for Clinical Pastoral Education.

Byrd, R.C. (1988). Positive therapeutic effects of intercessory prayer in a coronary care unit population. *Southern Medical Journal, 81*, 826-29.

Fitchett, George et al. (2000). Spiritual Care in the Hospital: Who Requests It? Who Needs It? *The Journal of Pastoral Care*, Vol. 54(2), 173-186.

Salzman, M. (2000). *Lying Awake*. New York: Random House, Inc. p. 179.

Shakespeare, Wm. (1957). *The Merchant of Venice*. NY: Simon & Schuster, Act 3; SC 2, 49.

Southard, S. (1976). *Religious Inquiry*. Nashville: Abingdon Press.

VandeCreek, L., Bender, H., & Jordan, M. (1994). *Research in Pastoral Care and Counseling*. Decatur, GA: Journal of Pastoral Care Publications Inc.

Ministry for the Good of the Whole

Eugene W. Huffstutler, DMin, BCC

SUMMARY. Clinical pastoral education and professional chaplaincy have long struggled with their relationships to various scientific worlds. With others, I affirm that the Emmanuel Movement, which produced unprecedented collaboration between clergy and physicians, died because its leaders failed to grow, to continue collaboration, and to train other physicians. I describe various indicators that suggest an increasing rapport between pastoral care and the sciences. *[Article copies available for a fee from The Haworth Document Delivery Service: 1-800-HAWORTH. E-mail address: <docdelivery@haworthpress.com> Website: <http://www.HaworthPress.com> © 2002 by The Haworth Press, Inc. All rights reserved.]*

KEYWORDS. Ministry, chaplaincy, clinical pastoral education, science

As the question of whether Clinical Pastoral Education (CPE) and chaplaincy ought to become more scientific is joined, two points of clarification are necessary. First, the linking of CPE and chaplaincy has long been assumed and in some instances, this is helpful. However, in this instance, it may serve to blur lines of responsibility deriving from

Eugene W. Huffstutler is affiliated with The McFarland Institute, 1400 Poydras Street, Suite 936, New Orleans, LA 70112 (E-mail: ghuffstutler@tmcfi.org).

[Haworth co-indexing entry note]: "Ministry for the Good of the Whole." Huffstutler, Eugene W. Co-published simultaneously in *Journal of Health Care Chaplaincy* (The Haworth Pastoral Press, an imprint of The Haworth Press, Inc.) Vol. 12, No. 1/2, 2002, pp. 99-102; and: *Professional Chaplaincy and Clinical Pastoral Education Should Become More Scientific: Yes and No* (ed: Larry VandeCreek) The Haworth Pastoral Press, an imprint of The Haworth Press, Inc., 2003, pp. 99-102. Single or multiple copies of this article are available for a fee from The Haworth Document Delivery Service [1-800-HAWORTH, 9:00 a.m. - 5:00 p.m. (EST). E-mail address: docdelivery@haworthpress.com].

10.1300/J080v12n01_11

clarity of mission. Also, the Association for Clinical Pastoral Education has already chosen to become more "scientific" by adopting educational outcomes into its Standards (ACPE Standards, 2002). This step, required by the United States Department of Education accrediting process, was a major factor in the disaffection of a highly vocal ministry within ACPE who claimed that by becoming more objective, ACPE had lost its soul.

This issue tends to prompt that kind of response, represented by a kind of moral urgency, if not self-righteousness. The origins of CPE in the United States were marked by a similar division between two groups who differed primarily in their response to the emerging science of psychodynamic theory (Thornton, 1970). ACPE history also yields lessons relevant to our current situation. Thornton suggests that the Emmanuel Movement, which produced unprecedented collaborations between clergy and physician, died because of the failure of its leaders to grow, to continue collaboration, and to train other clergy.

We currently possess a similar opportunity for growth or failure. The Interfaith Health program at Emory University (2001), for example, recently published an open letter suggesting the following signs of convergence between health (medical science) and faith:

- A stream of research now explores how spirituality affects individual health outcomes as a protecting and coping factor. Even more promising research is emerging concerning the roles of faith structures and their capacity to contribute to community health.
- Changes in Federal policy such as "charitable choice" are increasing the direct funding of religious-based projects involving key health issues that are also increasing the attention to how we evaluate and hold accountable these efforts.
- It is now common for health initiatives involving behavioral risks such as HIV, substance abuse, and violence to work closely with community based religious groups. This large body of knowledge is being carefully reflected upon.
- Nearly every national religious body has developed training and education units focused on health for its members and as ministries for others. Thousands of congregations now have staff and volunteers working in these areas.
- The health sciences are increasingly interested in social determinants of health and community-based initiatives, which is opening a new era of examination into the complex role for religion and religious structures in society.

The letter goes on to suggest more research, new competencies, and more collaboration.

The scene is not unlike 1987, when Elizabeth McSherry, MD and William Nelson, PhD, posited that the DRG era was an opportunity for increased pastoral input, if not a crisis of survival. McSherry advocated a new clinical science of chaplaincy that excited some and repelled others. Yet, her naming of the DRG crisis for chaplains as one of survival proportions was entirely accurate. Further, her most controversial suggestion, namely that chaplains make notes in patient charts, is now commonplace.

One would hope that research demonstrating the efficacy of pastoral care would likewise become commonplace. A recent publication (O'Connor, Meakes, Davis, Koning, McLarnon-Sinclair & Loy, 2001) suggests that it is not. Efforts to produce studies that sustain patient-centered spiritual care ministry are more encouraging. As VandeCreek and colleagues (2001) suggest, "The health care chaplaincy profession lacks information to address important questions about their activities" (p. 297). Why? They suggest, "This lack of information may reflect a tendency on the part of professional chaplains to be concerned only with their own departments and situations rather than the profession as a whole" (p. 297). Such a narrow vision will ultimately limit professional chaplaincy.

I believe that the basis of professional chaplains' identity is as trained theologians. Further, the contemporary understanding of culture, provided by social sciences, requires a contextual theology (Bevans, 1992). While contextual theology can be carried out in a number of ways, all require taking the context of ministry seriously. Whatever else might be said of the setting for professional chaplaincy today, knowing the language of science and business is a requirement. Whether one does translation of theological concepts into this language, points out theological themes inherent in this language, or pays attention to action and the meaning one may infer from that action–all are appropriate approaches. It is inappropriate to ignore the scientific and business context in which many chaplains do their work.

Those who resist becoming more scientific have at least one point, however. As Douglas John Hall (1996) suggests, the church (translate chaplains) is a ministry that exists for the good of the whole. It is unable to do so, though, unless it retains its essence–its uniqueness. It is easy to be tempted by the power that medical science and business seem to offer. It is helpful to remember that even when speaking in the "foreign language" of science or business, chaplains have a representative role. The chaplains' presence represents the presence of the transcendent. In some sense, becoming more "scientific" or "business-like" may just "pay the rent" so that we can do our essential work as theologians and remain those who represent the involvement of the Holy in affairs of persons.

REFERENCES

Association for Clinical Pastoral Education, Inc. (2002). *The Standards of The Association for Clinical Pastoral Education, Inc.*, Decatur, GA: ACPE, Inc. 9-11.

Bevans, Stephen B. (1992). *Models of Contextual Theology.* Maryknoll: Orbis Books, 7.

Interfaith Health. (Fall, 2001). *Faith and Health.* Emory University.

Hall, John Douglas. (1996). *Confessing the Faith.* Minneapolis: Augsburg Press, 119-134.

McSherry, E. & Nelson, Wm. (1987). The DRG Era: An Opportunity for Increased Pastoral Input, or a Crisis for Survival? *Journal of Pastoral Care*, XLI(3), 201-213.

O,Connor, T., Meakes, E., Davis, K., Koning, F., McLarnon-Sinclair, K., & Loy, V. (2001). Quantity and Rigor of Qualitative Research in Four Pastoral Counseling Journals. *Journal of Pastoral Care*, 55(3), 271-281.

Thornton, E. (1970). *Professional Education for Ministry.* Nashville: Abingdon Press, 23-99.

VandeCreek, L., Gorey, E., Siegel, K., Brown, S., & Toperzer, R. (2001). How Many Chaplains Per 100 Inpatients? Benchmarks of Health Care Chaplaincy Departments. *Journal of Pastoral Care*, 55 (3), 289-303.

Chaplain Yes and Chaplain No:
Both Are Correct; Neither Is True

Steven S. Ivy, PhD

SUMMARY. This article supports chaplain investment in research activities. These activities should be guided by recognition of the complexity of human experience, integrative theologies and philosophies, and systemic consciousness. *[Article copies available for a fee from The Haworth Document Delivery Service: 1-800-HAWORTH. E-mail address: <docdelivery@haworthpress.com> Website: <http://www.HaworthPress.com> © 2002 by The Haworth Press, Inc. All rights reserved.]*

KEYWORDS. Chaplaincy, spiritual care, research

Empirical attention to the actions and effects of spiritual caregivers is by no means a new enterprise. Numerous Biblical accounts (e.g., I Kings 17; II Kings 5; Luke 8:41-52; Acts 14:8-10) report the physical effects of prophets and healers on those to whom they minister. The case study method has been an effective teaching tool for clergy throughout the twentieth century. For over one hundred years social scientists such as William James and Gordon Allport have studied spiritu-

---

Steven S. Ivy is Vice President for Values, Ethics, and Pastoral Services, Clarian Health Partners, Inc., Indianapolis, IN 46206-1367 (E-mail: sivy@clarian.org).

[Haworth co-indexing entry note]: "Chaplain Yes and Chaplain No: Both Are Correct; Neither Is True." Ivy, Steven S. Co-published simultaneously in *Journal of Health Care Chaplaincy* (The Haworth Pastoral Press, an imprint of The Haworth Press, Inc.) Vol. 12, No. 1/2, 2002, pp. 103-112; and: *Professional Chaplaincy and Clinical Pastoral Education Should Become More Scientific: Yes and No* (ed: Larry VandeCreek) The Haworth Pastoral Press, an imprint of The Haworth Press, Inc., 2003, pp. 103-112. Single or multiple copies of this article are available for a fee from The Haworth Document Delivery Service [1-800-HAWORTH, 9:00 a.m. - 5:00 p.m. (EST). E-mail address: docdelivery@haworthpress.com].

10.1300/J080v12n01_12

ality in a variety of physical and social contexts. What is relatively new is physicians utilizing the standard research tools of their discipline to study the possible effects of spiritual practices and cultures on the physical health of individuals and cohorts (Larson, 1998). The argument between the two chaplains presented earlier in this volume results in an interesting question: What is the proper place of the scientific method in shaping spiritual ministry?

A Hasidic story tells of the wisdom of both journey and home. It is a long story, but a summary will suffice here. A rabbi lived in a poor village that had no resources for proper education of the children. He lived in great angst about this. He had a series of dreams in which he went to a distant city, looked under a bridge, and found great wealth. After the third repetition of the dream he undertook the journey, found the bridge and searched under it, but to no success. He was about to depart in even greater angst when a soldier who had been watching him asked what he was up to. The rabbi told the soldier his story. The soldier scornfully replied, "You stupid old man, I too have had a dream three times in which I went to a poor village, looked under the stove of the school, and found a horde of money. You do not see me making that kind of journey just because of a silly dream." The rabbi bowed low, returned to his school, dug up the floor under the stove, found the money, and built the finest school in the entire region.

As with all such teaching stories there are multiple layers of meaning. This article will explore the purpose of spiritual caregivers' interaction with the "unknown" and how it allows chaplains to "return home" with a deeper truth. To that end, this article will argue that each chaplain is correct in the positions each holds; also, each does not quite state the truth.

WHAT IS THE PROBLEM?

The rabbi is clear; the children need an education. Both chaplains agree that spiritual care is an important technology for ministry and also agree that this technology should remain available to persons through the healthcare delivery system. But their definitions of the problem to be addressed are quite different.

The research-affirming chaplain defines the problem as–healthcare reform is based upon evidence-based medicine. No one wants to pay for any cost within their healthcare bill that does not contribute to their well-being. If it is to remain a viable department within evidence-based healthcare practice, chaplaincy must demonstrate that it has positive effects so that healthcare managers have objective reason to include it in their budgets. Thus, chaplains should produce science that reflects their value to the healing environment. (Of course, the actual practice of medicine is far from this standard. The Office of Technology Assessment (1994) reports that up to 80% of medical interventions are based on the clinical expertise of the practitioner rather than an empirical knowledge base.)

The research-avoiding chaplain defines the problem as–spiritual care contributes to the well-being of patients in ways that are not dependent upon scientific measures of knowing. Adopting the scientific method may result in two problems. First, the paradigms of knowing between science and religion are different. Thus, to use the research methods of science to demonstrate the value of faith will distort one, if not both domains. Second, if chaplaincy adopts scientific methods and does not prove its validity through these methods, chaplains will not have a place in the healthcare budget. Thus, chaplains should remain within their tradition of developing sustaining relationships and practices that are valuable, regardless of their effectiveness as measured via scientific methods.

Both of these perspectives appeal to the same core concerns–ministry, science, and business. They each do so in a way that dichotomizes ideals and focuses on self-protective role consciousness. In order to move beyond their dichotomy, chaplains must adopt a broader understanding of their work environment and their ministry. A brief review of three perspectives from employee coaching, philosophy of science, and business may assist in moving beyond the dichotomy.

A VOICE FROM EMPLOYEE COACHING

One dimension of healthcare reform focuses on the work environment itself. As with most work environments, its over-arching characteristic is increasing complexity. Nowhere is that more true than in healthcare. All employees are increasingly required to take on multiple roles, to act with individuated autonomy that benefits the institution, and to maintain a high degree of self-consciousness (Kegan, 1994). Even though chaplains' CPE experiences are based upon a self-directed learning theory, many (most?) find moving to a truly autonomous yet systemically connected style of ministry very difficult. Kegan describes key demands of the modern work life and offers several suggestions. Among the more illuminating to the chaplains' conflict are:

- Be accomplished masters of your work roles and your careers.
- See the organization from the "outside in"; see your role in relation to the parts and the whole. (p. 302)

This perspective suggests a place to stand in relationship to the conflict between the chaplains. Chaplains are already conscious of being in complex relationships. The notion of being "betwixt and between" is certainly not new (Holst, 1985). Yet the insecurity of that position continues to trouble chaplains. In the present context, chaplains are asked to provide evidence of their pragmatic value; yet, they represent traditions of long and sustained value. The healing institution to which chaplains tie their vocations is tied to research; how can chaplains escape similar accountability? The healing institution to which chaplains tie their vocation is also tied to finitude, chance, and chaos; how can chaplains forsake the deep knowledge of needed spiritual response? An accomplished master must be well versed in both the art and theory of a profession. Since science is one base of theory and religion is the other, chaplains cannot avoid responsible engagement with research.

Thus, one response to the debating chaplains is, "You must move beyond the either-or debate. What will help you act responsibly to the multiple audiences you serve–patients and families, hospital staff, medical care providers, your spiritual and religious sponsors?"

A VOICE FROM PHILOSOPHY

The philosophy of science focuses on the epistemological question: "How do I know what I know, and, how can I demonstrate that it is true?" (Hamlyn, 1967). Some affirm intuition and others insist on sensory experience as the key to knowing. Some appeal to the logical superiority of "the true" while others claim the value of (or the superiority of) "the beautiful" or "the good." Ian Barbour (2000) has developed a four-fold model for examining the ways in which science and religion have sought resolution of these differing perspectives. He names these modes: conflict, independence, dialogue, and integration. Each of these models is suggestive of ways in which chaplains can encounter research in order to enhance spiritual care.

The key philosophies representing a "conflict model" of interaction are scientific materialism and Biblical literalism. Materialism holds that matter is the fundamental reality of the universe. Scientific materialism holds that the scientific method is the only reliable method to know the truth about that matter. This philosophy may claim that the only actions that really matter are those that affect the physical body and the only way to know the effect of one's actions is through the classic method of scientism, a double blind, placebo controlled, randomized trial. Most medical research is grounded in this philosophy. In settings where the transcendent is excluded and the spirit is marginalized, research into the spiritual dimension of human experience is a nonsequitur at best. Thus, the research-avoidant chaplain wants nothing to do with research.

Biblical literalism represents the belief that all truth worth knowing is revealed through scripture. Scientific research may be accepted as long as it does not conflict with a tenet of faith; if it does, it must be rejected. For example, the creationist certainly accepts the science that draws oil from wells, converts it to gasoline, and powers his car. But he will reject the science that describes the processes of creating the oil as requiring millions of years. Medical care has long abandoned the practice of operating from revealed truth. Thus, the research-approaching chaplain wants nothing to do with a stance that appeals to revealed authority and common practice as its base.

The "integration model" of interaction between science and religion seeks to deepen both science's and religion's capacities for interpenetrating the reality of the other. It moves toward a post-modern resolution of the divergence of science and religion. The search is for a deeper synthesis that yields a more profound understanding of reality. Both natural theology and process philosophy are examples of an integrative style. Natural theology will have a more transcendent emphasis while process philosophy will likely have a more immanent emphasis. They are joined in the search for a comprehensive metaphysic that is inclusive of both known scientific knowledge and technological perspective. Examples of integrative methods include Michael Polayni (1946, 1958) on "personal knowledge" and various process philosophies. Wilbur (1998) developed a contemporary example of philosophical and psychological integration called Great Holarchy–the unity of sense, reason, and spirit.

The chaplains could each find a productive stance within this method. The research-approaching chaplain could focus on the questions of health and healing while maintaining contact with more material science colleagues. The research-avoidant chaplain transforms the objection into a creative question. This chaplain could focus on ensuring that the deep questions and answers of spirit are included in both design and result of any significant studies.

A VOICE FROM BUSINESS

Healthcare reform is not only an issue of science. In fact, the greater issue may well be economic reform. In the United States sickness care and health care constitutes the largest single component of commerce, 13.4% of the Gross National Product annually (Millenson, 2001). Thus, the discussion of what constitute "knowledge" (and thus responsible practice) has large economic consequences. This is even more true in an environment in which costs are rapidly increasing and pressures to restrain costs are growing. Thus, "health care reform" may refer more directly to financial concerns than to medical practices that increase well-being.

Seventy years ago the costs of sickness care were paid by individuals and supplemented by the charitable impulses of religious groups and local taxpayers. Physicians and nurses thought primarily of their vocations as service. Today costs are paid by complex insurance and tax systems (although individuals are being given increasing responsibility for direct payments). Physicians and nurses may think more of career than of service. Of course, the chaplains' paradox is directly related to these changes. Seventy years ago hospital chaplaincy was in its infancy and spiritual care was primarily a function of churches and church associations. Today it is a semi-autonomous profession dependent upon the budgets of medical systems for financial sustenance. Chaplains' professional and financial ties are more invested in their hospital than in their religious community or judicatory.

The mission and values of hospitals, those who own and govern them, the payers, and the patients are undergoing rapid and exceedingly complex change. The anxiety that is always a correlate of change is represented by the conflict between these chaplains. One seeks to secure a place through a knowledge route not usually associated with religious ministry while the other seeks security through an appeal to authority that is greatly separated from the day-to-day reality of most healthcare systems.

DIRECTIONS FOR ACTION

The rabbi acts in accord with his passion; he builds a school. Chaplains must participate in the journey to experience the common ground of the empirical and the transcendent, the sensory and the spiritual, the interior and the exterior, as they are found in health care (Wilber, 1998).

This passion is not about reforming the healthcare system in the United States. It is not about proving our value as ministers. It is not about proving that spirituality does make a difference in health outcomes. Rather, the journey is one of developing wisdom, relationships, and focus. It is about continually drawing attention to the importance of the whole person as the subject and object of physical and spiritual attention. In the process chaplains may contribute to a reformulation of the fundamental mission, values, and vision for spiritual-relational-physical care.

The unifying theme latent within these disparate voices is that contemporary professional life is complex. It demands that each profession and each individual within that profession creatively engage those perspectives that are different, especially those which break previous models of thinking and perceiving. Scientific methods of research may accomplish this, but they may also bind to a particular worldview. Systematic questioning is to be valued by chaplains, scientists, and hospital spirit-keepers. What are some specific avenues that can be formulated? The following prescriptions offer directions for exploration.

First, chaplains should be aware of the spiritual problem constructed into some research. Some of the current research in spirituality and health subsumes spiritual practices under the rubric of therapeutic modality. Thus medicine becomes the controlling metaphor and prayer or forgiveness (or other practice) becomes a technology for health. "Complementary medicine" modalities are faced with the same dilemma. They hear the message, "Give up your other-than-scientific paradigm, submit your practices to empirical verification, and then you may be admitted to the practice of care" (read "insurance reimbursement and hospital-based practice").

Chaplains should be very cautious participants in such endeavors. For example, prayer effectiveness studies are deeply flawed when they are based in a non-theistic cause-effect paradigm. Such studies ignore a core foundation of all theistic prayer claims; it is not the prayer or the pray-er who causes a change, but a gracious God (Cohen, Wheeler & Scott et al., 2000). The soul of medicine and the medicine of the soul would benefit more for spiritual care research to focus on how spirituality adds to the coping capacity of patients. "Considering the ways to bring medicine closer to a recognition of (the importance of spirituality) would be more beneficial than applying the scientific method to prayer" (Chibnall & Jeral, 2001; 2535).

Second, chaplains should generate scientific research that allows knowing to include more than empirical evidence. Studies that include dimensions of beauty and good as realms of knowledge would be valuable contributions to the literature. Spiritual care leaders should assist in studies in which music, art, poetry, and dance are included in the treatment regimen. Where empirical evidence can demonstrate these as healing, so be it. But the more important concern is how these modalities of experience contribute to persons' purpose, meaning, and well-being. For example, what is the role that spirituality, faith, and religion play in interpreting crises of meaning in the face of acute illness, accident, and chronic disease? Measures of whether those who have access to faith actually experience less costly medical procedures are of little interest in that which really matters (Chibnall & Jeral, 2001). Technology is not the ultimate mediator of reality and physical health is not the ultimate goal of life. Chaplain research must help contextualize the technological.

Third, spiritual care providers should develop and participate in studies that attend to the ethical and spiritual climate of institutions and caregivers. For example, in some hospital systems professional ethicists (either philosophically or medically trained) have displaced spiritual leaders as ethics leaders. Clinical and biomedical ethics have forgotten that their roots include a strong stream of religious contributions. Chaplains can reclaim the importance of this endeavor for interdisciplinary leadership. An excellent example of such a thought leadership is David Guinn's work (2001) that articulates the ethical foundations of complementary medicine. He demonstrates the importance of adhering to both the roots and the future of a perspective rather than simply adapting to another's worldview. In a similar manner, chaplains' leadership in ethics "adds value" to the business of healthcare.

Another productive question might focus on the effect of chaplains leading efforts to build "spirit in the workplace." Ministry to staff has always been considered an essential hallmark of chaplains' role. Chaplains have attended to this through individual relationships and through providing the rituals of the faith traditions. Within the field of spirituality studies there is a strong upsurge of interest in Celtic Spirituality. Within the field of business there is a strong upsurge of interest in spirituality. Both of these emphasize finding God in the midst of the everyday, anywhere and everywhere. Chaplain research in workplace spirituality would further both business and spiritual agenda.

A third question might focus directly on the ethical: Do spiritual practices and beliefs impact health care decisions (Cohen et al., 2000)? Research in this area would gain insight into how patients exercise their decision-making autonomy, how they feel supported, and how they maximize their sense of well-being. Again, it would be integrative in that it would seek to understand persons as integrated persons.

CONCLUSION

This article has argued that chaplaincy must become more scientific. But that stance must be rooted in an integrative philosophy, not a materialistic or literalistic stance. The nature of the modern hospital and the expectations of the business that employs chaplains both move the profession toward such a stance. Nevertheless, the motivation for this practice must grow from self-defined, self-evaluating, and progressive intentions.

Those who provide spiritual care through the medical care system have a dream. The dream requires a difficult journey. In the midst of the journey chaplains must not lose sight of their core truth. The real treasure is at home. The real treasure is the wonder of the human person in relationship to community and to God.

REFERENCES

Barbour, Ian (2000). *When Science Meets Religion.* New York: HarperCollins.

Chibnall, John & Jeral, J. (2001). Experiments on distant intercessory prayer. *Archives of Internal Medicine,* 161, 2529-2535.

Cohen, Cynthia, Wheeler, S., Scott, D. et al. (2000). Prayer as therapy: A challenge to both religious belief and professional ethics. *Hastings Center Report,* 30 (May-June 2000) 40-47.

Guinn, David E. (2001). Ethics and integrative medicine: Moving beyond the biomedical model. *Alternative Therapies.* 7, 68-72.

Hamlyn, D. W. (1967). History of epistemology (Vol. 3) *The Encyclopedia of Philosophy.* New York: Macmillan 9-38.

Holst, Lawrence E. (1985). *Hospital Ministry.* New York: Crossroad.

Kegan, Robert. (1994). *In Over Our Heads: The Mental Demands of Modern Life.* Cambridge, MA: Harvard Press.

Larson, David B., J. Swyers, & M. McCullough. (1998). *Scientific Research on Spirituality and Health: A Consensus Report.* Rockville, MD: National Institute for Healthcare Research.

Millenson, Michael L. (2001). *Hospitals and Health Networks/IDX 2002 Digest of Health Care's Future.* Chicago: Health Care Forum.

Office of Technology Assessment. (1994). *Identifying Health Technologies that Work: Searching for Evidence.* Washington, DC: U.S. Congress Office of Technology Assessment.

Polayni, Michael. (1946). *Science, Faith, and Society*. Chicago: University of Chicago Press.

Polayni, Michael. (1958). *Personal Knowledge: Towards a Post-Critical Philosophy*. Chicago: University of Chicago Press.

Wilber, Ken. (1998). *The Marriage of Sense and Soul: Integrating Science and Religion*. New York: Random House.

Language and Tools
for Professional Accountability

Mark E. Jensen, PhD

SUMMARY. The article considers the issues raised by Chaplain Yes and Chaplain No earlier in this volume. They are considered in the framework of the distinctive dimensions of a profession. I contend that chaplaincy could be served by internal discussions of specialized skills and goals it wants to claim in the professional sphere, and that scientific tools could be used to evaluate, refine, and communicate those skills and goals. Possibilities include benchmarks, outcomes research, and inclusion of "consumers" in research designs. I argue that distinctive core skills and competencies of chaplaincy lie in affective, intuitive, and symbolic domains more than scientific domains, but that chaplaincy can benefit from strategic utilization of tools more native to other disciplines. I caution against reductionism from either domain, while arguing for vigorous dialogue. *[Article copies available for a fee from The Haworth Document Delivery Service: 1-800-HAWORTH. E-mail address: <docdelivery@haworthpress.com> Website: <http://www.HaworthPress.com> © 2002 by The Haworth Press, Inc. All rights reserved.]*

Mark E. Jensen is affiliated with Wake Forest University Baptist Medical Center, Department of Pastoral Care, Medical Center Boulevard, Winston-Salem, NC 27157-1099 (E-mail: mjensen@wfubmc.edu).

[Haworth co-indexing entry note]: "Language and Tools for Professional Accountability." Jensen, Mark E. Co-published simultaneously in *Journal of Health Care Chaplaincy* (The Haworth Pastoral Press, an imprint of The Haworth Press, Inc.) Vol. 12, No. 1/2, 2002, pp. 113-123; and: *Professional Chaplaincy and Clinical Pastoral Education Should Become More Scientific: Yes and No* (ed: Larry VandeCreek) The Haworth Pastoral Press, an imprint of The Haworth Press, Inc., 2003, pp. 113-123. Single or multiple copies of this article are available for a fee from The Haworth Document Delivery Service [1-800-HAWORTH, 9:00 a.m. - 5:00 p.m. (EST). E-mail address: docdelivery@haworthpress.com].

10.1300/J080v12n01_13

KEYWORDS. Chaplaincy, pastoral care, clinical pastoral education, science

Early in 2001, professional organizations representing five groups of spiritual care providers approved the final draft and subsequent publication of *Professional Chaplaincy: Its Role and Importance in Healthcare.* While not the first, last, or exhaustive word on the subject(s), this document represents some important new ground in the cultural and professional discussions about healthcare and spirituality. First, the collectivity of these diverse professional organizations aimed at modest consensus advocating for the importance of spiritual care in the provision of health care. Second, and more germane for this discussion, it attempted to utilize empirical, quantitative studies in arguing the case.

As one of the writers of this "white paper," I have heard and read various reactions to it. "There is not a prophetic word in it," an officer of one of the organizations declared to me. A letter in the *Journal of Pastoral Care* (Keese, 2001) contended that the paper appealed to the "baser instincts" of both the culture and the professional organizations. These criticisms, and others like them, let me know that despite approval from the boards of our organizations, the internal professional discussions were far from over. One hopes they have at least begun.

I've listened also to the reactions from 'outsiders' who have read the paper. One group, mostly business people, told me they never knew chaplains did so many different things. They thought chaplains prayed and came when people died. A scientist and administrator cited it in a paper he wrote for a professional society. Interestingly, what he cited were two images from the first section of the paper. The first image was taken from a poem by Wendell Berry (1994) entitled "A Parting." The poem describes an old farmer who, in his old age, has come "into the care of doctors, into the prison of technical mercy." The second image comes from an article written by Gibbons and Miller (1989), in which they argue that health care institutions risk becoming "biological garages" if they do not tend to the deeper dimensions of personhood. The scientist quoted the least scientific parts of the paper. The business people quoted the most concrete and descriptive dimensions of the paper.

Perhaps what is unique to the paper is that it combines the analogical with the quantitative and discursive. Some readers found the quantitative to make plain what they could not discern by casual observation or from chaplains' previous attempts to tell the larger world what we do. Others found the analogical (images) giving voice to intuitions for which they had not previously found language. The native skills and core competencies of chaplains are probably more like the poet's than the scientist's, and engaging this discussion will move both groups considerably out of our comfort zones of professional expertise.

What persons in the care of both chaplain and scientist seem to be saying is that they need the skills of both to be cared for well. What spiritual care providers and those of us who train them need to grapple with is whether, and to what extent, we need to utilize the methods of the scientific community in the pursuit of excellence in training and care. In this article, I organize my contribution to this discussion into some contextual observations, some implications for chaplaincy, and some implications for chaplaincy education.

THE CONTEXT OF THE DISCUSSION

I note several things about the context in which these issues are being discussed. These factors will continue to influence the shape of the questions and possibilities for collaborative responses.

First, alternative and complementary therapies have marched from the margins to the mainstream. Therapies that would not have been near academic medical centers are increasingly common within their walls. Insurers are covering a growing range of these therapies, or offering their subscribers discounts. These decisions have been driven largely by consumer demand, not by scientific study. Many of these alternative and complementary therapies involve, either implicitly or explicitly, practices, disciplines, or cognitive belief structures from a variety of spiritual and wisdom traditions. In other words, investigations in complementary therapies are leading directly to questions and investigations regarding spirituality.

Second, accrediting agencies now recognize spiritual care as essential to health care, and mandate it as a patient right. Definitions and elaboration of standards related to spiritual care are only in their infancy. What will our input be into their development?

Third, cultural interest in 'spirit' and 'soul' is present everywhere. Check out the titles in everything from the religion section to the financial planning section of bookstores, actual and virtual. The interest in spirit and soul extends into leadership and management theories and corporate values and culture. Translating such cultural trends can be tricky business, but this observer sees culture hungry for mythic, narrative, and spiritual meaning alongside the technical and rational.

Fourth, technological advances in medical care are not slowing down. Digital technologies are making possible non-invasive imaging, diagnosis, and treatment either in radically miniaturized or virtually non-invasive forms for a variety of medical ailments. Genomic studies hold enormous promise for understanding and treating a whole range of ailments. Interest in "non-scientific" alternative therapies does not imply that scientific advances and questions are not major forces in healthcare's future.

Fifth, there are only so many minutes, so many dollars, and so much need. How do we decide what is the most effective, the most affordable, and the most pressing? The rationalization and commodification of health care continue. Institutions demand revenue, payers demand evidence of effectiveness or reduced cost, and consumers demand access to the whole range of possible therapies. Can spiritual care continue to avoid participation in or definition by these movements? It is at this point that the critics of the White Paper mentioned above aim their best intentions, fearing capitulation to the language and forces of the market at cost of heart, soul, and unique identity.

Sixth, spirituality, sometimes defined in ways that involve professional chaplains, and sometimes in ways that do not involve them, has become a hot item in healthcare research. Chaplains have been involved in, and major contributors to, some of this literature. Those professional chaplains who have contributed on the empirical side of these conversations are not large in number, and generally received their training for such participation on the run or outside conventional ministry/chaplaincy education. The studies getting the most comment currently are experimental studies on the effects of prayer, variously and tortuously defined. While a variety of research designs mark the field, the most influential and numerous studies involve quantitative designs and correlative statistical methods. The prayer studies mark the movement from simply correlative analyses to experimental designs, where patients are randomized to one "treatment," another treatment, or no treatment. Note that few of these studies, correlative or experimental, look to psychodynamic traditions for their theoretical home. To the extent that chaplains and CPE supervisors still rely on that broad tradition and its methods, the newer collaborations leave us out of the one branch of human "sciences" (one corner of psychology) where we felt most at home. While psychodynamic theory-building flourishes in some places, it would not be an overstatement to say it is increasingly seen as a marginal voice in theological and psychological worlds, both academic and clinical.

I venture some summary comments on these contextual observations. First, the taboo about dealing with religion in health care is gone. It is increasingly permissible to speak of religious/spiritual things in the medical context, and to study them. Medical researchers are studying them the best way they know how, using methods with which they are familiar. Unless and until we demonstrate the utility of alternative methods to investigate these questions, quantitative (scientific) methods will dominate the discussions. Second, there are simultaneous movements in seemingly contrasting directions. Some movements in health care are toward further technical and scientific modalities, and some movements are toward affective, intuitive, mythic, ritual, holistic, religious modalities of care. In other words, professionals and consumers are moving in scientific and seemingly non-scientific directions at the same time. Perhaps it is only professionals trained in one mode or another who experience these movements as confusing or contradictory. Another way of describing these movements in several directions is that we are seeing the possibilities and dilemmas of a postmodern era, where no single 'paradigm' holds complete sway over the cultural, theoretical, or clinical landscape.

Finally, one of the ways to interpret this consumer-led charge into alternative models of treatment (that includes a new openness to spirituality) is as protest against a health care system that, at its worst, deprives them of voice, and fails to attend to the issues of conflict, value, meaning, and patients' inner worlds in the quest to cure disease. Spiritual care providers ought to heed this protest, and see one dimension of our task as helping patients find voice to construct, preserve, and transform meaning and significance in the experience of illness. The work of Arthur Frank (1995), for instance, makes this case eloquently. Frank defines the need for ill persons to find voice as a postmodern ethical conundrum and imperative.

The remainder of this article develops my notions that chaplaincy in health care settings can both benefit and contribute by making limited and focused use of some methods considered more "scientific," while staying rooted to our core competencies. I contend that the concerns raised by Chaplain Yes and Chaplain No more accurately concern how chaplains will engage the larger processes of professional accountability and multidisciplinary dialogue. The final section suggests parallel implications for training done by the Association for Clinical Pastoral Education.

STAKING A PROFESSIONAL CLAIM: CHAPLAINCY

Camenisch (1991) suggests that a profession has at least four distinguishing marks: (1) specialized skills and knowledge; (2) professional autonomy; (3) a distinctive goal; (4) motivation outside personal gain. The question of what methods chaplains should use to advance knowledge and practice should flow from how we respond to at least the first and third elements of professional functioning: the skills we claim and the goals of our work. If we claim expertise in spiritual care, and if we can name the distinctive goal(s) of our work in spiritual care, then we can move to consider what methods we use in advancing knowledge and evaluating effectiveness.

Clarifying our particular skills and goals is a discussion that has internal and external dimensions. We cannot look to other professions to tell us what our primary skills and goals are; in an important way, this is an internal discussion. The nature of professional functioning, however, is staking that claim in a public sphere with other professionals and the persons whom we serve. In clarifying our primary skills and goals internally, we would do well to speak our most native language. Translating those claims in the public sphere involves the work of translation, and quantitative language is often the *lingua franca* of interdisciplinary discussions in health care.

In translating for the various public spheres, we will not want to give up our native tongue, nor fail to recognize where translations into the tongue and methods of science and commerce are crude and inadequate. The subtleties of any language system can only be appreciated by immersion in it. That implies that some professionals in both religious/spiritual and scientific domains will need to risk the learning curve of immersion in the other's language. What professionals in both domains are right to resist is becoming a subset of the other. Conversely, the "internal" and "external" work of the various professions can be enriched by genuine dialogue.

In spiritual care, quantitative methods can help establish benchmarks and study outcomes in the service of the professional goals we claim. Debate about the appropriate benchmarks can proceed accordingly. VandeCreek, Siegel, Gorey, Brown, and Toperez (2001) published a study measuring chaplains per 100 inpatients as a proposed benchmark for institutional strategic planning and evaluation. Our department has begun utilizing another benchmark in our attempts to improve quality. For the last two years, we have had in place a re-designed process for keeping statistics on our ministries. Clearly not a perfect process, it has given us some new ways of evaluating our efforts. One of the "benchmarks" we have begun to monitor is something I have called the "coverage fraction." The coverage fraction is defined by taking the total number of hours our department spends in ministry on a designated patient care area and dividing that total by the number of patient days for the same area. The resulting fraction is the hours per patient per day our department spends in various ministries to that unit. By comparing the fractions, we have been able to identify units that appear to be "overcovered" or "undercovered relative to the mean for types of patient care areas." When we begin asking why, at times we discover there are good reasons. At other times we discover we need to allocate our time and efforts in different ways. These two benchmarks are examples of descriptive statistics. They merely give us better language to describe and understand what it is we are doing. As such, they can help us move toward standards for adequate provision of spiritual care.

Comparing outcomes through the use of correlative statistics is another use of quantitative methods. Similar to benchmarks, outcome studies can help the internal and interdisciplinary discussions of skills and goals claimed by our profession. For example, is reduced length of stay an outcome chaplains want to embrace as intrinsic to our professional practice? Patient satisfaction? Neither of these things seems to be harmful. If they are negatively correlated in some instances, what would we understand the goal of spiritual care to be, and what outcomes would signify excellence in pursuit of that goal?

George Fitchett's recent work (1999) moves in the direction of correlating spiritual distress with various patient outcomes. One of the good things about Fitchett's work is that it moves toward correlating outcomes with assessments that flow more clearly from spiritual care language. Fitchett's work also advances the discussion about how to make good assessments, and what outcomes chaplains are most likely to be able to effect. Continued discussions of spiritual care goals and patient outcomes will both benefit from and contribute to research correlating spiritual care and patient outcomes.

As we design and participate in these studies, what are the standards of care that guide us? "Standard of care" becomes an important way to enter into research using quantitative measures, particularly of experimental design. Clinical trials of new drugs, for example, are rejected if any of the subjects of the study intentionally receives less than what is considered standard medical care for their condition. Are we ready or able to begin defining standards of care for various subject populations? If so, will we use divisions of subject populations that follow medical assessments, or will we group subjects from assessments that follow from our understanding of spiritual care? Is it ethical, for example, to prospectively randomize patient groups to receive no professional spiritual care? If they would receive professional spiritual care without the research design, I would argue that we can not endorse or participate in such a design.

Various consumer health and activist movements have begun to have impact in advocating for patient inclusion at all levels of research: selection, design, and evaluation (Wiliamson, 2001). As chaplains continue to make progress in research and research design, why not invite "consumer" collaboration in the discussion of research priorities and design? Chaplains could empower patients and learn about research that matters to them by inviting and designing patient collaboration in spiritual care research. Such a move would combine concerns about patient empowerment, research ethics, method, and design.

I believe that well-conducted research will help us achieve some of what I hope to communicate to medical colleagues about the religious and spiritual dimensions of human beings, and which unsophisticated understandings of religion and spirituality fail to grasp. I find myself trying to find ways to communicate to my medical colleagues a number of things their training has not automatically prepared them to understand:

- Religion is more than belief.
- Religion and spirituality are amazingly diverse and multidimensional.
- We've only begun to understand the complex relationships between spiritual practices, consciousness, and physical systems.
- Our individual orientation in western culture (and medicine) has led us to overlook and fail to appreciate social and community dimensions of spirituality and religion, and our research designs demonstrate this one-sided focus.

Well-designed descriptive studies in spiritual care will, I believe, continue to demonstrate these and other things in ways that health care, including spiritual care, may be able to understand and utilize. Chaplains ought to help design and participate in these studies. No study starts from a theoretical vacuum, and our theories about the nature of the spiritual life can and should inform quantitative designs.

I contend that one of the sets of specialized skills and goals around which chaplains should claim specialized expertise is as midwives of the human capacity for making meaning. Claiming our expertise in this way will, no doubt, disappoint some who would want more explicitly religious or theological ways of staking our claim. At the same time, it will remind us and our colleagues from other disciplines that our effectiveness is not measured by exactly the same set of patient outcomes as is an experimental drug or treatment trial. Translating such a claim into quantitatively tested methods will yield a variety of possibilities, none of which will completely capture or translate the heart of the matter, but all of which could help us describe and evaluate what it is we do. Chaplaincy has little to lose and much to gain from participation in well-designed quantitative studies. Having said that, it is time to cut the question down to size. Methods are properly seen as tools for larger purposes. The tool should fit, and not change the purpose of the one using it. As long as identity and purpose are clear, chaplains need not fear such methods, even if we feel intimidated by them. Similarly, we need not abandon or apologize for other tools with which we are more adept: idiographic, qualitative, phenomenological. In fact, we should use them and be clear about their strengths and practicality. A recent article by O'Connor et al. (2001) makes it clear that spiritual care publications make only marginally better use of rigorously conducted qualitative research than quantitative methods.

IMPLICATIONS FOR CHAPLAINCY EDUCATION

Having argued above that utilizing quantitative methods can help chaplains' elaboration of specialized skills and goals, I venture a few observations about implications for education done by Association for Clinical Pastoral Education centers. It should be noted that ACPE, Inc., Standards (2001) have already begun moving toward clearer articulation of outcomes, coming in part out of the accreditation process with the U.S. Department of Education. While few certified pastoral educators likely believe that these outcomes exhaust the meaning, or even adequately describe the core of what they hope for in their educational efforts, they provide statements that help educator and student be accountable to one another and to the process in which they are engaged. The work of identifying and clarifying outcomes in the training process will, and no doubt should, continue.

But what are the implications of this discussion for our core competencies? Do the questions raised in this collection of essays, or the notions I have about how to respond, bear on what we should be aiming for and evaluating as core competencies for chaplains? Should chaplains become routinely competent in designing or interpreting quantitative studies in health outcomes? Probably not. I would argue, in parallel fashion, that physicians should not become routinely competent in taking a spiritual history or doing a complex assessment for spiritual care. There are simply other things at the heart of the profession for both physician and chaplain that require rigorous and sustained attention. Nevertheless, some chaplains would do well to pursue at least minimum competency in the language and methods of empirical research. We would do well to identify research collaborators who are more skilled in the complexities of these methods when we utilize them. We may need to find ways to nurture chaplains who choose to specialize in research as part of Level II specializations and beyond.

Spiritual care research does suggest some interesting directions for chaplain competencies. As one of the foci of spirituality and health research is spiritual practices (the most common being prayer and meditation), chaplains need to develop some minimal competencies in leading a variety of spiritual practices and disciplines. Chaplain assessments should move toward identifying with whom and when these practices might be indicated and contraindicated, and begin helping health care teams understand these subtleties.

Another implication of the language of outcomes and the further clarification of core competencies comes in the designing of CPE curricula, particularly residency curricula. This is where collaboration between the professional certifying bodies and clinical education programs is crucial. In our center, for example, we have begun thinking that a two-year residency ought to bring one to the competency level to be certified as a Board Certified Chaplain by APC. Thus, in designing curriculum, we have begun to place ACPE outcomes and APC standards for certification alongside one another to guide us. Our hope is to construct a framework of accountability between our professional organizations, our students, patients, families, staff, and ourselves. None of these sets of documents is perfect. None of them say all I'd like them to say, nor do I pretend they fully communicate what it means to do quality spiritual care. That is hoping far too much for the kind of language they require.

CONCLUSION

While spiritual care tends to meaning and mystery, we cannot simply retreat to the language of mystification if we would be colleagues to other professionals, and if we would serve well patients, families, and staff. Conversely, searching for one-to-one correspondences between languages of science and spirituality is to fail to recognize the strengths and limits of either. That does not mean we should despair of the dialogue.

A reductionist reading of either spirituality or science by the other is a dead end. Knowing how many cycles per second is in a particular note is important for standardizing the building of musical instruments and the apparatus to tune them. Yet, that knowledge cannot communicate what happens when an artist plays a well-crafted melody on a precisely tuned instrument. Musicians know that precise tuning and inspired melodies are both important, even though one cannot account for the other.

Scientific language and method are a language of precision. Religious language and ritual are languages of symbols, which by their nature are not as precise and measurable. Humans seem to be wired for both languages. Physicians and chaplains will lose nothing by learning and appreciating what they can about the language of the other. To my mind, explorations in the language of precision cannot help but clarify and renew, while never replacing, the language of the heart.

REFERENCES

Association for Clinical Pastoral Education, Inc. (2001). *Standards.* Retrieved December 21, 2001, from <http://www.acpe.edu/acroread/standards01.pdf>.
Berry, W. (1994). A Parting. *Entries: Poems by Wendell Berry.* NY: Pantheon Books, 11.
Camenisch, P.F. (1991). Clergy ethics and the professional model. In J. Wind et al., *Clergy ethics in a changing society.* Louisville, KY: Westminster-John Knox Press.
Fitchett, G. (1999). Selected resources for screening for spiritual risk. *Chaplaincy Today, 15(1), 13-26.*
Frank, A.W. (1995). *The wounded storyteller.* Chicago, IL: The University of Chicago Press.
Gibbons, James L. & Miller, S.L. (1989). An Image of Contemporary Hospital Chaplaincy. *Journal of Pastoral Care, 43*(4), 355-361.
Keese, P. (2001). Letter to the Editor. *Journal of Pastoral Care, 55*(3), 328-329.
O'Connor, T.S., Koning, F., Meakes, E., McLarnon-Sinclair, K., Davis, K., & Loy, V. (2001). Quantity and rigor of research in four pastoral counseling journals. *Journal of Pastoral Care, 55*(3), 271-280.
VandeCreek, L., & Burton, L., eds. (2001). A white paper: Professional chaplaincy: Its role and importance in healthcare. *Journal of Pastoral Care, 55*(1), 81-97.
VandeCreek, L., Siegel, K., Gorey, E., Brown, S., & Toperez, R. (2001). How many chaplains per 100 inpatients? Benchmarks of health care chaplaincy departments. *Journal of Pastoral Care 55*(3), 289-301.
Williamson, C. (2001). What does involving consumers in research mean? *Q J Med, 94,* 661-664.

Four Fatal Flaws
in Recent Spirituality Research

Raymond J. Lawrence, DMin

SUMMARY. The answer to the question of whether clinical pastoral education and professional chaplaincy need become more scientific should be a Tillichian "yes and no." Pastoral care and counseling is both an art and a science. The field is thus subject ineluctably to scientific examination. However, its artistic dimensions are elusive and impenetrable to scientific scrutiny. *[Article copies available for a fee from The Haworth Document Delivery Service: 1-800-HAWORTH. E-mail address: <docdelivery@haworthpress.com> Website: <http://www.HaworthPress.com> © 2002 by The Haworth Press, Inc. All rights reserved.]*

KEYWORDS. Chaplaincy, spirituality, science, research

Religion is generally similar to art in that it appeals largely to the arena of feelings, imagination, and values, bearing an elusive power to move and inspire people. What in one generation appears to be significant and powerful sometimes appears in the next to be pap. We do not know how to measure scientifically the differential power of Hamlet,

Raymond J. Lawrence is Director of Pastoral Care, New York Presbyterian Hospital, Columbia Presbyterian Center, and General Secretary, College of Pastoral Supervision and Psychotherapy (E-mail: lawrenr@nyp.org).

[Haworth co-indexing entry note]: "Four Fatal Flaws in Recent Spirituality Research." Lawrence, Raymond J. Co-published simultaneously in *Journal of Health Care Chaplaincy* (The Haworth Pastoral Press, an imprint of The Haworth Press, Inc.) Vol. 12, No. 1/2, 2002, pp. 125-130; and: *Professional Chaplaincy and Clinical Pastoral Education Should Become More Scientific: Yes and No* (ed: Larry VandeCreek) The Haworth Pastoral Press, an imprint of The Haworth Press, Inc., 2003, pp. 125-130. Single or multiple copies of this article are available for a fee from The Haworth Document Delivery Service [1-800-HAWORTH, 9:00 a.m. - 5:00 p.m. (EST). E-mail address: docdelivery@haworthpress.com].

http://www.haworthpress.com/store/product.asp?sku=J080
10.1300/J080v12n01_14

125

Walt Disney, Harry Potter, or of Bach, the Beatles, or rap music. The capacity of science to penetrate and evaluate them is quite limited. How would we weigh the relative truthfulness, therapeutic effectiveness, and values of a Jonathan Edwards, Billy Graham, Mahatma Gandhi, Pius XII, or Anton Boisen? Each was effective religiously speaking, but each is quite different from the others. All are appropriately subject to critique, but an evaluation process will be largely subjective and intuitive. Thus a thorough scientific assessment of the truth, therapeutic power, or values of the various manifestations of religion is an impossible assignment.

On the other hand, certain aspects of religious functioning can certainly be measured scientifically, such as, for example, the quality and nature of interpersonal communication skills. All religious practice depends on interpersonal communication, and communication can be measured and tested in scientific ways, and the quality and type of communication, whether primary process or secondary process, can be assessed. One might even say that the quality of interpersonal communication ought to be measured and evaluated scientifically in those proposing to offer pastoral care and counseling. Professional respect in a clinical setting would seem to demand as much. Thus we could say that there needs to be more of this kind of scientific examination of chaplaincy and pastoral counseling services.

The foregoing is hardly the stuff of controversy. And yet current high-profile scientific study of religious and pastoral practice in a medical context is touched by significant controversy and tainted by a widespread, and, I believe, appropriate malaise in the religious and scientific communities. The principal point of controversy is the challenge made to the bulk of spirituality and prayer research of the past decade, a challenge thrown down to claims that data demonstrates the efficacy of prayer to effect healing. The principle spokesman for the debunkers of these research results is Richard Sloan (1999; 2000) who contends that current research is for the most part faulty, and that it does not measure up to the accepted standards of scientific research. His arguments are persuasive, and his conclusions are a troubling commentary on the state of discourse between medicine and religion. That so many reputable persons in both religious and scientific communities would endorse what may be patently faulty data in an eagerness to promote religion is a remarkable phenomenon of our times. It suggests, among other conclusions, a high degree of anxiety on the subject.

Sloan's (1999; 2000) critique of recent research is a purely scientific one, speaking as he does from the perspective of a research psychologist. However, the research of the past decade is also tainted by critical theological and philosophical problems. I propose that four fatal flaws taint recent efforts to apply scientific analysis to the practice of religion in the health care field, and more particularly recent scientific research into the efficacy of prayer in the healing process.

First, the presumption that God can be scientifically researched is a fatal flaw in recent religious research generally. It is so faulty a position in fact that it is laughable. Only this world and creatures in this world can be researched. Any other worlds that may exist are at present unavailable to scientific scrutiny. That this point has to be made to the scientific community is in itself passing strange.

The presumption that God can be researched is never stated boldly, but it is typically implied. For example, when the various research protocols enlist monastics and prayer circles in various religions in order to test their effectiveness, they are implicitly testing God. God is presumed to be an actor in the communication interplay. The presumption is that God responds to the pious and devout of the recognized world religions. No research reports have surfaced yet of tests that use, say, a similar group of stockbrokers or computer programmers or voodoo practitioners. The assumption is that God would be less likely to turn an ear and take action on behalf of such a group. Thus has prayer and spirituality research slipped obliquely into undertaking scientific examinations of God's actions.

This error could have been avoided if researchers would have adopted what could be called "the letters to Santa Claus model" in prayer research. It goes like this: As raw data, letters written to Santa could certainly be researched. Such letters might provide data about attitudes toward giving and receiving, for example, and reveal information about the attitudes, values, and character of young children. Collaterally, parents might also benefit from their children's letters, revealing what is on their minds. The research might discover that writing to Santa is therapeutic in some manner. It might even discover that children who write to Santa have an 11 percent lower mortality rate. But if research into letters to Santa were to slip into promoting a belief about the actions of Santa himself, and reach conclusions about which letters Santa is more likely to answer, it would have overreached itself, and crossed the boundary between the arena of science and the world of imagination.

God may be the name of a reality more real than Santa, or maybe not, but the research problem is the same. In the final analysis research cannot deal at all with Santa himself or God per se, but entirely and exclusively with human phenomena and nothing else. For research purposes

God must be relegated to the realm of Santa, as having no researchable existence, the status of a product of human imagination.

Second, recent scientific research implicitly implies that spirituality is one thing, and particularly one benign thing. This is misleading because spiritualities are legion. So many varied and divergent spiritualities exist representing the most wildly contradictory values that to speak of spirituality as if it is one thing is to make oneself unintelligible. That so much of the current research assumes that spirituality is one benign unexamined entity is evidence of an absence of a critical faculty that one does not usually expect from scientists.

Hardly any religious tradition supports the notion that among all the many gods of the world, one is as good as another, an implicit premise of contemporary research on religion. One of the seductions of the recent fad of multiculturalism is the pretense that one God is as good as another.

Provocative though such a contention will be, I argue that no one should presume to speak on the subject of spirituality unless prepared to discourse on the spirituality of Adolf Hitler and Nazism. Among 20th century political figures, Hitler had few equals in presenting himself as a spiritual leader. He revived the spirit of the German people humiliated and shamed by the defeat in World War I and more so by the terms of the Versailles settlement. Hitler's statue among Germans in the late 30s was exceedingly high, a consequence of his restoring their sense of pride. Furthermore, Hitler publicly proclaimed his belief in God and his belief that God had appointed him the task of reviving the German people. When news came to Hitler in his bunker that Roosevelt had unexpectedly died on April 12, 1945, Hitler, himself having only two weeks to live, told his entourage that Roosevelt's death was a sign that Providence was changing the course of the war (Kershaw, 2000). The fact that Hitler was a cruel and sadistic tyrant does not disqualify him from the attribution "spiritual." If we can parse the spirituality of Hitler and Nazism we demonstrate that spirituality may have a positive or negative valence.

The many and varied spiritualities of the world and of history require critical scrutiny. Even within particular religious organizations or creedal groups that have strict dogmatic boundaries we can observe a wide range of spiritualities. For example, striking variations of spirituality are evidenced in three randomly picked modern Roman Catholic popes: John XXIII's all-embracing, earthy humanity and openness to the world at large, the stingy, ascetic, introverted coldness of Pius XII, and the worldly ruthlessness of Pius IX who kidnapped a young Jewish boy and kept him for pederastic purposes (Cornwell, 1999).

Any discussion of spirituality carries with it an implied, if not explicit, set of values. Any discussion of spirituality that leaves the implied values unexamined is a discussion without substance. Any scientific examination of spirituality in any form must know the character of the spirituality on which it focuses. Current research generally takes a naively uncritical stance toward the spirituality that it tests for results. It is a fatal flaw.

Third, current research in the field of spirituality and medicine is generally pursuing the wrong material. The question of whether 500 nuns praying for a particular suffering individual have potency to effect improvement in the health of that individual is a relatively uninteresting question. The efficacy of such a prayer lobby, were it to be demonstrated as efficacious, would only prove something in the arena of parapsychology, in the realm of mind over matter, or some new law of physics in the sensory-kinetic field. While such a scientific discovery would be useful, it is also mechanistic and impersonal, and is far removed from the heart of religion. In that sense recent research pursues the chaff rather than the wheat.

Paul Scherer (1960), the late Lutheran preacher in New York, solved the problem of the efficacy of prayer playfully but soundly, theologically speaking. He pronounced that all prayer is answered. Most of the time, he said, the answer is "no." Scherer's simple rejoinder undermines the theological validity of recent prayer research that takes no account for the "no."

Current research on prayer has focused entirely on intercessory prayer, an inflation of one specific type of prayer above all others. In most religious traditions intercessory prayer does not predominate. It is only part of a larger understanding of prayer that includes adoration, repentance, and thanksgiving. The motivation for the focus in recent research on intercessory prayer is clear. It hopes to find a lever whereby religion might become another instrumentality for implementing our wills to overcome our fate. If such an instrument could be found, we would of course all use it. However, the discovery of such an instrument to control our destiny is by definition outside the boundary of most of the so-called "higher religions."

Recent research has reduced successful prayer to one in which our wishes are accomplished. Theologians such as Paul Tillich, on the other hand, calls a successful prayer one in which the Spirit speaks through our spirit, which is to say, a prayer in which we are grasped emotionally and intellectually in a profound way and given a new perspective on life.

Fourth, the fourth fatal flaw in much recent scientific research into the effectiveness of religion is that it displays theological illiteracy. Scientists who do research on religion are obliged to have read the basic literature, or at least to use consultants who have studied the subject. For example, Harold G. Koenig (1999) writes on the subject of the justice of God, an age-old theological problem referred to as theodicy. Koenig boldly declares that illness is not punishment from God, and that God's work is that of healing. Koenig does not betray an awareness that he has bitten into an ancient and troublesome theological and philosophical problem that he presumes to solve in the most cursory manner. Even Woody Allen demonstrates a more profound awareness of the problem when he says that God is just, but simply an underachiever.

Koenig and his colleagues are actually promoting a new, banal theology. He promotes a God who is a benign, doting father who wants everyone to be content and happy with as little effort as possible, a God whose character structure is similar to that of the U.S. Congress, attending to whomever has the loudest voice and the most money. Koenig, and others like him, are theological naifs who pose as world experts on religion. His recommendation of the pious religious publication, "Guidepost," is further evidence of his cursory review of theology.

We need more scientific study of religion and religious practices. But current research generally is profoundly flawed, and if Sloan is correct, it is flawed both scientifically and theologically.

REFERENCES

Cornwell, J. (1999). *Hitler's Pope*, New York: Viking Press.

Kershaw, I. (2000). *Hitler: 1936-1945 Nemesis*. New York, W. W. Norton & Co., p. 791.

Koenig, H. (1999). *The Healing Power of Faith: Science Explores Medicine's Last Great Frontier*. New York: Simon & Schuster.

Scherer, P. (1960). Union Theological Seminary (Richmond) class.

Sloan, R., Bagiella, E., & Powell, T. (1999). Religion, Spirituality, and Medicine, *Lancet*, 353: 664-667.

Sloan, R., Bagiella, E., VandeCreek, L., Hover, M., Casalone, C., Hirsch, T., Hasan, Y., Keger, R., & Poulos, P. (2000). Should Physicians Prescribe Religious Activities? *New England Journal of Medicine*, 432: 1913-1916.

In the World but Not of the World: Going Beyond a Dilemma

Richard Leliaert, OSC, PhD

SUMMARY. Is the issue addressed in this volume a question like "What time is it?" or a Quest-ion like "What is time?" I argue that it is a quest-ion that requires professional chaplaincy to quest for an answer although it will always have blurred edges that lack succinctness, clarity, and certainty. The challenge posed by the quest-ion means that we must transform the dilemma into a higher synthesis that respects the qualitative aspects inherent in the profession. *[Article copies available for a fee from The Haworth Document Delivery Service: 1-800-HAWORTH. E-mail address: <docdelivery@haworthpress.com> Website: <http://www.HaworthPress.com> © 2002 by The Haworth Press, Inc. All rights reserved.]*

KEYWORDS. Chaplaincy, pastoral care, research, science

The question before us is quite focused: Should clinical pastoral education (CPE) and professional chaplaincy become more scientific in response to healthcare reform? My first thought is to ask: Is this a question

Richard Leliaert is Manager, Spiritual Support Services, Oakwood Hospital and Medical Center, Dearborn, MI 48123-2500 and Chairperson of the Board, National Association of Catholic Chaplains (2001-2003) (E-mail: Leliaerr@oakwood.org).

[Haworth co-indexing entry note]: "In the World but Not of the World: Going Beyond a Dilemma." Leliaert, Richard. Co-published simultaneously in *Journal of Health Care Chaplaincy* (The Haworth Pastoral Press, an imprint of The Haworth Press, Inc.) Vol. 12, No. 1/2, 2002, pp. 131-141; and: *Professional Chaplaincy and Clinical Pastoral Education Should Become More Scientific: Yes and No* (ed: Larry VandeCreek) The Haworth Pastoral Press, an imprint of The Haworth Press, Inc., 2003, pp. 131-141. Single or multiple copies of this article are available for a fee from The Haworth Document Delivery Service [1-800-HAWORTH, 9:00 a.m. - 5:00 p.m. (EST). E-mail address: docdelivery@haworthpress.com].

10.1300/J080v12n01_15

(like 'what time is it?') or a quest-ion (like 'what is time?'). I don't think the above question can be answered clearly and simply like 'what time is it?' It's more a quest-ion, that is, we need to quest for the answer, and no matter what answer(s) we provide, there's always that blurred edge that doesn't provide the succinctness or clarity or certainty we'd like. Try answering the question, "What is time?" If we provide a 25 word or less answer, it can never encompass the depth and breadth of the question (Stephen Hawking not withstanding). So it's not a matter of good or bad questions, but a matter of a qualitative difference between the approaches taken by Chaplain Yes and Chaplain No.

With the publication of the White Paper titled *Professional Chaplaincy: Its Role and Importance in Healthcare* (2001), the focus question takes on much greater importance. Both the spiritual and professional dimensions of healthcare chaplaincy will be integrated and intertwined in the next millennium. So the responses of Chaplains Yes and No must be addressed and evaluated in the light of this reality. Chaplain No argues that CPE and professional chaplaincy will "lose their voice just when they need it most." Chaplain Yes answers, "Yes, they will find their voice just when they need it most." Both address legitimate concerns: Chaplain No argues for the autonomy of ministry in a way that protects it from scientific reductionism, i.e., a simple 'ministry is nothing but, say, psychological practice with a religious label.' Chaplain Yes argues for the need to validate the professional aspect of CPE and chaplaincy in a way that other professionals can understand and relate to.

Basically Chaplains No and Yes see the tension between the qualitative (i.e., transcendent) side of ministry and its ability to be expressed in quantitative (i.e., scientific) terms. This is a tension whenever scientific survey research tries to capture the essence of a person or group's response to a significant question. From my viewpoint, it would be a mistake to simply argue for one against Chaplain No or Chaplain Yes; but neither is it a simple quest-ion of one being as good as the other. Both in my view capture *essential* aspects of the question, but a satisfactory response to the question means both views must be transformed into a higher synthesis that respects the qualitative aspects inherent in the quest-ion.

These tensions affect other disciplines and institutions in analogous or similar ways. Physicians experience this tension when they consider medicine as both an art and a science. (For example, I met a woman in our coronary care intensive unit who presented with severe chest pain; yet she told me that it was a year ago to the day that her husband died. A wise physician would be attentive to 'the broken heart' of a grieving woman as well as to her painful physical heart: medicine as art and science). Again, healthcare institutions face the tension between their role as service providers and as a business. Medicine is an art and healthcare is a service; they wrestle, however, with the realities of medicine as a science and healthcare as a business.

I appreciate the opportunity to respond simply because I'm not all that clear about my own thinking in this matter. I've had six units of CPE and have been in healthcare chaplaincy for about fifteen years. To begin my quest for a more adequate response, I take an image from Chapter 17 of the Gospel according to John in the Christian Scriptures. Therein Christ speaks of his disciples/ministers being simultaneously in the world (vv. 11, 13-5, 18) but not of the world (vv. 9, 14, 16). Verse 6 somehow incorporates both sides of the in/of the world tension. Chaplain No emphasizes the latter side of the tension, Chaplain Yes the former. My intent is not to oversimplify, but to keep a healthy tension between the valid aspects of both positions, which need to somehow get beyond the tension through a kind of transformation that might allow us even greater creativity. A tall order!

I start with some reflections on my own experience. Earlier this year I had contact with a man terminally ill with cancer. His family stated that according to his religious (Baptist) beliefs/values, he wanted, well really needed, to be baptized before his death. Only baptism by full immersion would suffice. His healthcare providers thought, "There's no way we can do this!" But an enterprising nurse and physician suggested they immerse him in a large rehab tank. It took a lot of doing to accomplish this, but the family's pastor did baptize him by immersion. The man was so overwhelmed by this experience that he began to improve significantly right after his baptism, and, almost incredible to say, he was in fact discharged from the hospital and did quite well for a significant length of time. This unexpected outcome provides a sense of the intersection of the divine into the material experience–in the world but not fully of the world.

Briefly reflecting on this scenario, Chaplain No would certainly see it as an illustration of his/her concern. Chaplain Yes might be a bit more ambivalent, but the effort of an interdisciplinary team to meet a stated need of the patient, whether team members were religious or not, paid off in an outcome that was indeed food for reflection. Did the inner transformation following the baptism, according to the faith of the patient and his family, truly express itself in an unexpected physical or clinical change in the patient's condition? I don't mean a miracle in the formal sense, but what people often call "a wonder-full happening."

This reflects the 'in but not of the world' tension that integrates both sides. If Chaplain No used this as a subject of a CPE verbatim, his/her theological reflection would emphasize their understanding of the transcendent at work. But would Chaplain Yes see this as a scientific validation of the effectiveness of pastoral care? Further, in an era of healthcare reform, certain results like a lessened length of stay (LOS) and/or significant cost containment might please insurers, or HMO executives, or hospital administrators, with all welcoming the positive patient/family satisfaction scores. Well, a win-win situation for everybody!

Let me turn to another experience at this point. Our hospital's quality assurance personnel informed all the managers that our Spiritual Support Services Department had the highest score for patient satisfaction of all the departments for a recent month. It was quite a welcome surprise for us in spiritual care, perhaps even more surprising for all the other departments. Then a separate Press Ganey survey of patient loyalty (that is, whether one would return to our hospital) for the same month indicated that we were one of eight departments to exceed our target score.

What does this mean? Well, would this be an indicator of what Chaplain Yes means by a scientific validation of our effectiveness as a spiritual care department? We were shown by a properly conducted set of surveys that we had achieved a high level of effectiveness vis-à-vis our peers. This was not simply our desire or judgment, but an empirical or objective evaluation of the results of our combined ministry. Most probably insurers benefited from the likelihood that we had some impact on a shorter LOS for some patients. It gave a fair indication of our professional competence and standing for our role in the interdisciplinary team(s) with whom we worked. Some asked us, in earnest or in surprise, "What's your secret?" or, "How did you do so well?" All in all, we were confronted with a quantitative measure of our accountability to our departmental and hospital goals as spiritual care providers.

So to return to the question: Should chaplaincy and CPE become more scientific in an era of healthcare reform? Both vignettes above indicate to some degree that both Chaplain No and Yes are indeed correct in their primary focus. Both vignettes illustrate that complex interplay between the ministerial/spiritual (the 'not of the world' aspect) and the professional/scientific (the 'in the world' aspect). Both immanence and transcendence, if you will, had their due. In more spiritual terms, God's working in and through, yet ever over and above, the concrete everyday world. The divine element is present in the material experience.

But, such scores do not necessarily indicate any kind of direct correlation, say, between a spiritual intervention and an outcome. As VandeCreek noted in *The APC News* (September-October 2001), there are a lot of considerations in answering a question like "Does Praying For Patients Really Help?" The results of survey research conducted by prayer researchers would not deter Chaplain No from believing in the power of prayer imbued by faith. Prayer is fruitful, regardless of research results. Chaplain Yes might point to the results described in VandeCreek's article as evidence that Chaplain No has little real validation for her/his claims about the effectiveness of prayer. An insurer or administrator might point to such an article as their 'out' for eliminating spiritual care departments in a budget crunch.

On a more personal level, as a Catholic priest I anoint persons with the Sacrament of the Sick. I engage patients and families of necessity from a faith perspective. As James 5:13-17 and the Ritual proclaim, "The prayer of faith will save the sick person, and if they have committed any sins, their sins will be forgiven them." How might we scientifically demonstrate the effectiveness of the sacrament of the sick? As we'll see a bit further on, I don't have any certain way of proving or even disproving the effectiveness of the Anointing from a scientific point of view. Whether a scientific study would validate or disprove the intimate connection between the Sacrament and healing (not necessarily a cure), I enter the Sacrament as sacrament from the perspective of faith, period! Its effectiveness as a work of grace really cannot be measured scientifically. Yet as the above scenarios might indicate, we need not posit an either/or, but a both/and.

Basically Chaplain No and Chaplain Yes might be at a standstill in responding to the opening quest-ion. Each of them, looking at the other's position, could end up deadlocked. But can we just leave it here? To begin our way out of the impasse, I point out some aspects that we need to consider.

- The importance of correctly understanding Jesus' statement: "Seek/strive first for the Kingdom of God and (God's) righteousness, and then everything else will be added/given to you as well" (Matthew 6:33). This saying can apply not only to bodily needs, but spiritual or emotional needs as well. This will be briefly addressed further on.
- The reality of holistic health. Modern healthcare, whether healthcare personnel recognize it or not, sees every person/customer/guest/patient (whatever term we use) as com-

prised of body, mind and spirit. Each are integrally (i.e., holistically) connected, and programs like the Harvard Symposiums on *Spirituality and Healing in Medicine* most likely are more than passing fads. The word for 'peace' as wholeness in almost all of the world's major religions (i.e., shalom in Judaism, salam in Islam, Om Shanti in Hinduism) conveys a holistic understanding of the human person.

- The distinction between cure and healing. If spiritual interventions are always geared to the cure of the person, and the person is not cured, say, of a terminal illness, does this mean that the spiritual intervention failed? Not really. Healing, on the other hand, means a more holistic state of being, wherein a person is at peace or at one with themselves, with God or their view of a higher power, with their loved ones, and with the created world. In my baptism example, even if there hadn't been a cure, or at least a remission of the terminal illness, the baptism healed the man in the sense that he was at one with himself, with God, with his family, and with God's creation.

- The limitations of science. In healthcare, evidence-based medicine, for example, is seen as scientific. Yet articles in medical journals indicate that evidence-based medicine is not as objective or as certain as many might wish to think. Much comes down to the reality of what is this person's condition? What are the factors that make this person's case unique, even in the face of much theory and research? Or, how can science verify pain scientifically? Our Policy and Procedure on Pain Management here at Oakwood Hospital specifically states, "Pain is what the patient says it is." There are lab tests for diagnosis of diseases(s), but not for the verification of pain. Pain is both objective-subjective in nature.

With the above caveats in mind, let's start with Chaplain No and Chaplain Yes both appealing to moral obligation. As I see it, our primary moral obligation is not primarily to theological or scientific criteria, per se. Our primary obligation is to minister to the felt need of a patient and his/her family. Whether one is religious or not, whether I am explicitly religious or not in my ministry, meeting the need of a person (as he/she states their situation) is our primary obligation. Our moral obligation is not to proselytize, or to convert, or to sneak in religious/spiritual comfort, or even to provide 'spiritual fluff.' Our obligation is not always to do whatever is asked of us (some requests are just inappropriate) but to respond ministerially in a way wherein we are truly pastoral.

So it is the patient's voice and not our agenda as chaplains or CPE students that provides the focus.

In an era of healthcare reform, CPE programs need to adjust to new realities. For example, patients are often in and out of healthcare facilities much faster than formerly. Hence our ministry needs to be more focused, even if limited to one visit. We don't have time as chaplains or CPE students/residents to probe into a patient's family of origin (background), or to engage in depth in psychological analysis of a patient's condition.

As chaplains, our pastoral or ministerial role is primary. In my view, CPE needs to be as attentive to the P (pastoral) in CPE as much as to the C (clinical). The pastoral also demands more attention to the religious/spiritual and cultural diversity of our world.

Theological reflection is an important part of the Verbatim, and over the past few years I've noticed a decline in the quality and depth of theological reflection amidst those students taking CPE in my hospital setting. While I am not claiming that this decline is universal, personal and other peoples' experience has told me that supervisors lack the theological component at the expense of a heavy psychological approach to ministry. A healthy balance is the key. This is too complex an issue to be addressed in an article of this scope; let me say that I and others have addressed these concerns, and specifically Roman Catholic concerns about CPE, in Volume 20 of *The Journal of Supervision and Training in Ministry* (2000).

However, Chaplain Yes's concerns for the scientific (i.e., clinical) dimension, as I see it, are not to be taken lightly. Now might be the time to ask, what does scientific mean for Chaplain No and Chaplain Yes. Both assume a clear meaning for scientific, but neither states it. In a pastoral or spiritual setting, 'scientific' can't translate simply into the kind of lab research that characterizes the Human Genome Project, for example. Neither can it mean the kind of research that involves watching the behavior of rats or other animals. (Even medicine cautions against assuming that what works in animals will work in humans. Recently a genetic researcher reported drastic failures of cloning efforts, Dolly and other animals not withstanding.) Does scientific mean the emerging science of neurotheology that focuses on links between the brain and spirituality (Rause, 2001)? This is the kind of research done by Newberg, D'Aquli and Raust (2001) in their book *Why God Won't Go Away*.

Scientific could mean properly conducted survey research, as we discussed earlier. Or does scientific translate into greater professionalism?

Somehow I think Chaplain No and Chaplain Yes are at bottom speaking of differing attitudes regarding the trend toward the professionalization of chaplains (especially through certification). For me anyway, this is the heart of the question posed at the beginning. C1 defends those chaplains (and CPE personnel) who are ministerially competent but not professionally certified. "I don't need to be certified to do good ministry" (like many ordained ministers claim they don't need an MDiv or any theological degree for that matter). Chaplain Yes argues that in view of healthcare reform there will be greater need to be professional chaplains. Only these can claim to be 'scientific' in the sense that professional means they provide more than spiritual 'placebos'–whether through prayer, Scripture reading, sacraments, etc.

Let me risk saying that Chaplain No's concern for the primacy of the religious/spiritual/theological is valid. When a chaplain, whatever their religious and/or humanistic perspective, encounters a person, especially via request or referral, the person understands the chaplain to be there for their spiritual/religious concerns; they are not looking for a psychologist or a social worker.

Hence the chaplain must first seek the equivalent of the Kingdom of God, so to speak, in the sense mentioned above, whether or not this is achieved in specifically religious ways. Then everything else will be added. A fruitful spiritual or religious interaction does not depend per se at that moment on whether I'm professionally certified or not. The grace of God determines the outcome(s), whether I see an interaction as successful or not. Yes, I realize my theological bias here, but we all have a bias. A value-free chaplain and/or professional simply does not exist. Any one of us can give countless examples from our everyday experience just how wonder-full, mysterious and yet frustrating the ways of God actually are, especially in end-of-life situations. God does as much in spite of us as because of us, whether we're professionally certified or not. Rather than diminishing us, this perspective frees us immensely. The outcome simply isn't in our hands, almost all of the time. This is no excuse to avoid being proactive, of course, but a humble recognition that 'the best laid plans of mice and humans do go awry' or that God often exceeds our expectations. There is the 'not of this world' dimension to our work as chaplains.

However, having said this, I do acknowledge that Chaplain Yes's is right on target with the concerns that chaplaincy become scientific in an era of healthcare reform, with the understanding that scientific aligns with professionalism. Mainly, because we do chaplaincy 'in the world.' We cannot avoid this dimension. We are not islands unto ourselves, but allied with our peers on interdisciplinary healing teams. We need to communicate with them as professionals in a language our peers can understand about our ministry and our role on the healing team. Our peers are also expected to be certified in their fields, and we should not and really cannot take certification lightly. Furthermore, areas pertinent to the national accreditation by the Joint Commission require a professional stance. I recall a formal Joint Commission visit, and the surveyors were interviewing the coronary care team. Right off, the physician interviewer said, "Well, let's begin with pastoral care. How do you fit into this team and how do you define your role?" Professional charting was critical to my response because if it wasn't documented, it doesn't exist. (I quip, the new Descartes is not Cogito, ergo sum, but, documentatum, ergo est–it's documented, therefore it exists.)

The demands of being a professional became clear to me after September 11th. When the Red Cross, for example, implemented its SAIR program to work with people affected by airline disasters, only those applicants with the proper professional credentials were accepted for training. Furthermore, when HIPPA regulations go into effect in 2003, it will be important to distinguish professional staff chaplains from local clergy. The latter *may* be excluded at first from access to patient information/data, because of HIPPA, but the former, as part of a hospital-based healing team, would be exempt from exclusion; chaplains, in other words, since they chart and are part of the professional staff, would have access to appropriate patient information.

Basically Chaplain No and Chaplain Yes can find common ground, in the light of the above remarks on professionalism, if we remember that being professional includes being a professor of faith (not dogmas) as well as a certified professional. Being a chaplain makes one commit to being a 'suffering servant' (involved in the demands of Service First, in secular language), insofar as there is an altruistic or 'other directed' focus to the professions. Hence, in being primarily focused on our chaplaincy profession, we can wear whatever professional credentials we bear a bit more lightly. I might say, in doing our work, let your framed document(s) simply hang on the wall or rest on the desk. A quiet confident demeanor makes us a more potent channel of divine grace, rather than a "if you got it, flaunt it" kind of attitude. It is a gift to be professional in both a spiritual and secular sense. Such, I think, is a harbinger of the chaplain of the future.

Lastly, as the transforming element of the 'in the world, but not of the world' tension, I want to go out on a limb a bit, without cutting off the limb. The prime medical model of the latter 19th and the 20th centuries has been somewhat as follows: focus first and foremost on healing/curing the body; then the healing of the mind will follow in the sense of a greater peace of mind, and maybe as an afterthought, you might tack on the spiritual. In other words, in the body-mind-spirit triad, it clearly reads from left to right. However, what if this emerging 21st century might show us, even from a scientific point of view, that it's completely the other way around? What if the healing of the spirit is the real key to greater peace of mind that then flows into the healing, and hopefully, the cure of bodily sickness or illness? Yes, I'll be the first to recognize that this is problematic. But then, as Einstein (1954; McFarlane, 2002) so well professed, even the answers to the mysteries of science are revealed to us, more than they are discovered by mathematical formula. What if, and yes it's a fanciful scenario at present, Einstein was telling us more than we're ready to admit, even as chaplains and CPE trained professionals? Talk about paradigm shifts.

Lastly, my model for this potential transformation is my ongoing reflecting on Jesus' healing of the paralytic in Mark 2:1-12. There was a healing, but the process begins with the healing of the paralytic's wounded spirit (by the forgiveness of sins). Then comes the gift of a renewed mind and heart: I'm a new person. And almost as an afterthought, the reminder of physical healing. As a Catholic priest, this healing model has helped me reflect more deeply on the Sacrament of the Sick, the Anointing of the Sick, which in line with James 5 integrates the forgiveness of sins as a part of the holistic healing of body, mind, spirit (see also I Thessalonians 5:23). Other spiritual traditions and perspectives can respond to this in their own way. I'm only reflecting on my experience as a chaplain and Catholic priest, and why I think the question posed at the beginning needs our constant attention and dialogue. That's why I am glad I accepted the invitation to make a foray into this crucial area. If nothing else, it's made me think through where I'm at, as they say, and it's made me appreciative of my chaplain and CPE peers in this dialogue.

REFERENCES

Einstein, A. (translated and revised by Sonja Bargmann). 1954. *Ideas and Opinions.* New York: Crown Publishers, 36-53.

Leliaert, R.M. (2000). The Future of Pastoral Supervision: Transmural, Transcultural, and Transformative Challenges. *Journal of Supervision and Training in Ministry,* 20, 166-75.

McFarlane, T. (2002). *Einstein and Buddha: The Parallel Sayings.* Berkeley, CA: Seastone Press.

Newberg, A., D'Aquili, E., & Rause, V. (2001). *Why God Won't Go Away: Brain Science and the Biology of Belief.* NY: Random House.

Rause, Vincent (2001). Searching for the Divine. *Reader's Digest, December 2001, 140-5.* From *The Los Angeles Times Magazine* (July 15, '01).

VandeCreek, Larry & Burton, Laurel, eds. (2001). *Professional Chaplaincy: Its Role and Importance in Healthcare.* The Association for Clinical Pastoral Education et al.

VandeCreek, Larry. Does Praying for Patients Really Help? *The APC News, 4, 17.*

At the Poles Eventually
All You Get Is Cold

Chaplain Arthur M. Lucas, MDiv, BCC

SUMMARY. I argue that any choice for either science or religion can necessarily only disserve those in the care of professional chaplains. The present and future of professional chaplaincy lies with integrating the strengths of the scientific method and attention to outcomes into the service of our calling in faithfulness, presence, compassion, and process. *[Article copies available for a fee from The Haworth Document Delivery Service: 1-800-HAWORTH. E-mail address: <docdelivery@haworthpress.com> Website: <http://www.HaworthPress.com> © 2002 by The Haworth Press, Inc. All rights reserved.]*

KEYWORDS. Chaplaincy, research, science

Well, of course health care chaplaincy and clinical pastoral education should avoid temptation! The positions of Chaplain Yes and Chaplain No are comparably flawed. They are asking the wrong question. And asking the wrong question can never lead to helpful answers. They framed either/or questions from the midst of needful tensions and then

---

Chaplain Arthur M. Lucas is Director, Spiritual Care Services, Barnes-Jewish Hospital, Washington University Medical Center, St. Louis, MO 63110 (E-mail: AML2792@bjc.org).

[Haworth co-indexing entry note]: "At the Poles Eventually All You Get Is Cold." Lucas, Arthur M. Co-published simultaneously in *Journal of Health Care Chaplaincy* (The Haworth Pastoral Press, an imprint of The Haworth Press, Inc.) Vol. 12, No. 1/2, 2002, pp. 143-150; and: *Professional Chaplaincy and Clinical Pastoral Education Should Become More Scientific: Yes and No* (ed: Larry VandeCreek) The Haworth Pastoral Press, an imprint of The Haworth Press, Inc., 2003, pp. 143-150. Single or multiple copies of this article are available for a fee from The Haworth Document Delivery Service [1-800-HAWORTH, 9:00 a.m. - 5:00 p.m. (EST). E-mail address: docdelivery@haworthpress.com].

http://www.haworthpress.com/store/product.asp?sku=J080
10.1300/J080v12n01_16

they answered them well. The higher challenge is approaching from a both/and perspective.

The positions, however, of Chaplain Yes and Chaplain No equally belie our calling into a professional world composed of both an art and science. Any time we allow ourselves the luxury of standing solely at either pole we pay a price in terms of our faithfulness and the good of those we serve. In so doing we avoid the requisite tensions for giving adequate (much less good, and far from excellent) compassionate, effective person-to-person ministry. The willingness and ability to stand in the midst of many tensions are woven into the fabric of our very calling. We are strangers in a strange land, whether we are amongst our health care or our community clergy colleagues. Dr. Peggy Way, in her address at the 1999 National Meeting of the Association of Professional Chaplains, aptly and touchingly described us as people on the margins. While we need to put in to port from time to time, she reminded us, our place is at sea, with our faith and the kerygma in our little boats. So, when we go to either pole of art or science, process or outcomes, faithful presence or calculated push, we are serving is our own respite from the tension. And eventually that will only lead to growing cold.

Think of the good nurses, physicians, and administrators you know or have known. Set aside for a minute all those who are problematic and you would just as soon avoid. Think of the good ones. I am willing to wager a lot (and my United Methodist Bishop knows I don't wager at all) that every single one of them knows his or her role in giving health care for human beings is both an art and a science. They strive every day to do their best in the midst of the confluence of their knowledge, personhood, professionalism and compassion. They work hard to provide ever more precise care for the individuals entrusted to them. They are willing to attend to what they know, think, feel and believe as they make the best possible decisions in their care giving. They are willing to take the risks inherent in being responsible caregivers in a field that is amazingly unpredictable, even given the expectations of certainty from the general community. And they are able to continue to *be with* people in the midst of doing their best for them. There are many ways their roles can be easier by quieting any one contrary polarity within these dynamics. And they believe their care will probably be a bit diminished every time they do so. How can we be less and consider ourselves called?

When we resolve that core tension of art and science, in any of its many manifestations, to one polarity or another, we need to be aware we most often are doing so out of our own need, fatigue or fear. We do so rarely because the truth resides at the pole. Our own needs are honorable. We deserve care and respite too. In fully being there for others, however, every nuance counts. Wholly eschewing any dimension of our person or profession costs the patient/family something. Fully being there includes being both vulnerable and intentional. Fully being there includes being both open to surprise and accountably intentional. Fully being there includes remembering what others for whom we have provided care have graciously taught us and recognizing the dazzling uniqueness of the person now before us. Fully being there includes accessing the insights and skills our colleagues offer us face to face and in the professional literature and the courage to respond spontaneously in the moment. Fully being there means calling on the reflection we can use, either privately or with others, to learn from our own experience for applications "the next time" and decathecting so our next interaction is as clean as we can manage. Fully being there means prayerful, thankful meditation on the presence of the Holy in our own lives, both individually and communally, which can be narrowly framed as piety. And fully being there means the informed intentionality that comes from subjecting our ministry to rigorous inquiry, which can be narrowly framed as the scientific method.

Ultimately, the measure of our chaplaincy is not about us, even though the primary stuff of our ministry involves our personhood, our faithfulness our vulnerability, our will and our inter-personal abilities. The measure of our chaplaincy is ultimately about the vulnerable people who entrust themselves to our care. It is not about our own scrupulous practice as a person and pastor. It is about the impact our person will have (for the good or ill, whether we like it or not) for the healing, well being and growth of the other. It is not about our faith in the healing process. It is about the faith of the person across from us and the dynamic life of that faith in his/her healing, well being and growth.

This often means professional chaplains and clinical pastoral educators have a more intense and convoluted challenge than do our professional colleagues in health care or theological education. Good doctors, nurses, and administrators other means, other stuff than themselves for their unique contributions to others' healing and well being. They have tools (needles, test tubes, medications) and ways (surgeries, tests, budgets, bench-marks) outside themselves as the "instruments" of their care and profession. We have ourselves, our presence and our inter-personal processes. We also, in faith, have God's presence, but that is not for us to prescribe or pretend to control. It is an extra mind twister to be clear our main tools are person hood and presence while at the same time attending to interventions and outcomes. Abandoning the twist is possible if we are all about our process and not about the others' experience. It is also possible to abandon the twist if we believe we are all about the difference we make, devoid of attending to the role of who and how we are with. Being relieved of the challenge to accountability outside ourselves is possible if we are only answerable for our personhood and not for the differences our personhood is making in the healing and well being of others. Maybe for us pastoral folks it is rightly, unavoidably about both who we are and what differences we are making, including our processes and our outcomes, the stories and the data, our faith and our facts.

The faithful use of good science can communicate with us about the associations we think may be there between our being and our difference making. It cannot tell us more about God as an effective instrumentation for treatment. And it cannot tell us about the rightness or "adequacy" of any one's beliefs as a force for healing. But applying some scientific tools and methods, like qualitative and quantitative research, data analysis and peer review to our ministry and what comes of our ministry in terms of others' experience can tell us how to be more focused, maybe even precise, in our efforts to be there for specific, unique others. Used well they can tell us how to be aware of the differences we are making. Used well they can inform us about how to be more care-fully intentional in the combination of whom and how we are with the impacts we have. And used well they will certainly call us to new heights of accountability outside ourselves, both individually and professionally.

Done well and with hoped for good "results" will this give us a voice at the health care table and justification for our standing in the healing arts and places? Why should we care? We have a voice. We have a place at the table. We have standing. And we have had them for a while. If the question is, Will the scientific data force others to hear our voice, recognize our place and respect our standing, the answer is: (all together now) NO! My experience with superbly data driven folks is that they are indeed data driven until they are confronted with data that does not fit their model of reality, their mythology if you will. Then that data are suddenly unpersuasive. Pushing the point further into the minutiae of their supposedly data driven world view by reducing our ministry to numbers, narrowly constructed quantitative research with the measure dictated by other perspectives, is bad pastoral care research. And bad research eventually disserves everyone, most importantly present and future patients and families. And it still will be unpersuasive to those entrenched in a worldview constructed on different impressions often believed to be data.

Will eschewing the scientific and standing wholly on faithfully, availably representing the Transcendent force others to hear our voice, recognize our place and respect our standing? The answer is: (all together now) NO! And it should not. As Dr. Peggy Way pointed out (1999), we work in the new cathedrals. I do not believe we should be valued simply because we are who and what we are, and are there. Only once in my recollection has "I Am" actually served that role appropriately. We are in cathedrals where everybody comes-for hope, healing, and compassion-not to see the priests practice their religion, no matter whom you name the priests.

What if we act like we have a voice, a place and a standing? Then the question about the engagement of science or any other discipline is not about our selling or winning anything, because we already have what we can buy or win. Then the question turns on what allows us to better meet people where they are, how better to give voice, effect from our place and exercise our standing in faith to the Word, to the person(s) in our care and to ourselves. Used with discretion and assertion the methods and means of the health care science world can help us serve others faithfully.

Early in my ACPE CPE experience I was introduced to the idea that ACPE CPE brings together knowledge of self, theologies and the human sciences in an effective person-to-person ministry. I bought it. And while I think I have grown and the profession has grown in understanding what all those elements entail and imply, I must admit I can never figure out how "bringing together" what the human sciences have learned (about change, or development, or communication, or coping mechanisms, or the grief process, or whatever) is good for pastoral care but "bringing together" the processes, methodologies and rigor of the human sciences (qualitative research, quantitative research, data analysis, peer review) is bad. Adopting the belief system of the human sciences is an entirely, wholly different matter. Being able to engage what is beneficial to our servanthood without having to adopt the belief system seems entirely congruent with our mandate to be in but not of the world, including the health care and scientific worlds. Doing so can help us meet people where they are, be more care-ful in the differences we are making and more accountable to them for the very stuff and impact of our ministry with them. It can even help us meet people like doctors, nurses, administrators and even payors, where they are while still standing as who we are where we are. And if we do that well, in a way that conveys the personhood, faith, story, and journey of the people in our care in a way the other professionals can hear they find it easier to incorporate the spiritual dimensions into improving their own care of those people. I say that as much from experience over the last few years in the ministry in this hospital as I do from any conceptual framework.

For instance one of the chaplains in this Midwestern, quaternary care, teaching hospital discovered early in his hospital ministry and clinical pastoral education a deep passion for victims of violence, specifically violent victims of violence (VVOVs), those who come to our emergency department shot or beaten or stabbed and who are themselves caught up in a life replete with violence. He initially conducted a demographic study to see if his impression of who these folks are as a group was supportable by hard data or simply the reflection of the individuals who had the most effect on him. It turned out his impressions were supportably accurate. One point of his supportable impressions included virtually all having had a history in their childhood of being meaningfully connected with a faith community and that was not the case for years before their appearance in our ER. With a major grant from the Lutheran Charities Foundation in St. Louis, he was then able to pursue his further impression that if the VVOVs meaningfully reconnected with a faith community of their choice then their quality of life could be improved (measurable by a verified instrument) and they could be relieved of showing up in our ER shot, and/or stabbed, and/or beaten. He is now conducting a carefully constructed study to find out if that impression is supportable too. (So far, so good.) We have already observed changes for the better in how other (note the import of the word "other") ED staff and physicians understand and relate with all the victims of violence who come (or are brought) to us for care. Our chaplain has long been valued there by these other care-givers. Over the last few years they have also been enabled to learn a lot from him in these special cases. The methodology he developed for his ministry with violent victims of violence can be found in *The Discipline for Pastoral Care Giving* (2001).

Should he have stopped with being passionately present for these wounded and often hope-deprived people? Should he have simply run on the assumption his impressions were accurate and what he thought should be a way to improve their lives did indeed improve lives and do it because it felt right? Should he do so even when it meant some other care for some other people would go undone in the process? On what should he base his decisions about the gift of his ministry and calling? If the data does not support the hopes he has for the interventions he has developed and the changes he has seen in a few lives, should he walk away from these folks as a bad investment? To have his place should he turn to ED leadership to tell him how to profitably spend his time there? Has he sold out by having the curiosity, discipline and courage to risk the rigors available in "scientific method?" Has he sold out to big business health care because the help he thinks he can offer people in real need may also lead to lower costs for our hospital? Or is he using all at his disposal to deepen and sharpen his passionate servanthood?

I could repeat the above refrain for our chaplain who benefited from conducting research as she focuses more sharply on the capacity to hope in her ministry with lung transplant patients. I could repeat it for our chaplain who has benefited our ministry and that of our special care center for women and children living with HIV/AIDS with her qualitative research into the role of prayer as these women make decisions about taking their medications. I could repeat it for our chaplain currently conducting a combination qualitative and quantitative research project on the meaning and impact of ritual for the grief process of women who have suffered a perinatal loss. Has each abandoned their calling to be a living reminder of the Holy by pursuing what they have? Spend one hour with any one of them and I sincerely doubt that thought will so much as occur to you again about her/his chaplaincy. Should they abandon that calling to be better scientists? Or would that only make them ineffectual pastoral researchers? Sold out? Hardly! Extended themselves to learn and grow for their care of others? Every time!

We are indeed lost if come to believe the ground of our voice, place and standing in health care rests on shortened lengths of stay, increased margins, higher patient satisfaction scores, or whatever other statistics to which other professionals with other beliefs wish to reduce our contributions in order to value them within their models and mythologies. We have a chance to rise to the challenge of asserting ourselves from our own grounds if we understand those efforts as attempts to call us to some accountability and better understand our voice, place and standing-our own contributions. If we merely assert they are asking wrong and wrongful questions, we are not being faithful to our calling to meet where they, are both the apparently ill and the apparently healthy. It is at least lazy, perhaps pompous and maybe idolatrous to brush aside their asserted ways of knowing accountability. It is inadequate for us to simply assert that we should be trusted and valued because we are who we are ("I AM!"). It is up to us to assert how we contribute. In health care today that is one way to be in community, to be engaged in the processes of the team and institution as well as with those of the patients and families. Being in community and engaged with others is our way and it is risky, be the community that of the least of us, those in their darkest hour, our peers, or colleagues or our bosses.

If we practice science at its worst (retreat to the pole of reductionistic data) or symbolic presence at its narrowest (retreating to the pole of righteously pious practice) we all lose. The integration of knowledge, skills, accountability and methodologies from science into the faithful practice of professional chaplaincy and clinical pastoral education is a daunting, sometimes frightening challenge. The vulnerable people who come to our institutions for care, are in our community in need of care and for whom we have a calling and responsibility to be in ministry are worth it. What makes it possible is our faithfulness, our will and our community, God's good will and Grace.

The worthwhile challenges are about how best to give voice for the healing, well being and growth of the people in our care in our positions in health care from our standing in the grounds of the Transcendent. In that, drawing together the best from science and art can only be our friend.

REFERENCES

VandeCreek, L. & Lucas, A.M. (eds.). 2001. *The discipline for pastoral care giving: Foundations for outcome oriented chaplaincy.* N.Y.: The Haworth Press, Inc.

Way, Peggy. (February 27-March 3, 1999). Chaplaincy–A Profession of Faith For The Future. Presentation at the Annual Conference of the Association of Professional Chaplains.

But What Are We Trying to Prove?

David B. McCurdy, DMin, BCC

SUMMARY. Chaplaincy and Clinical Pastoral Education (CPE) in the health care setting can and should approach their ministries more scientifically, primarily by incorporating the methods and results of quantitative and qualitative research. Such an approach, however, should have a carefully considered rationale. Proponents of a scientific approach should avoid associating their advocacy with dubious notions of health care "reform." They should attend to the perceptions–and fears–that chaplains may have of "science" and research as these affect pastoral care. In particular, fears for professional and programmatic survival should be recognized for their potential to predispose chaplains either favorably or unfavorably toward a scientific approach. Ultimately, chaplains should increase their openness to scientific methods in order to learn more about their ministry and improve their practice, without expecting that the adoption of research methods will be a magical solution to the problems posed by the current environment. *[Article copies available for a fee from The Haworth Document Delivery Service: 1-800-HAWORTH. E-mail address: <docdelivery@haworthpress.com> Website: <http://www.HaworthPress.com> © 2002 by The Haworth Press, Inc. All rights reserved.]*

David B. McCurdy is Editor and Research Associate, Park Ridge Center for the Study of Health, Faith, and Ethics, 211 East Ontario, Suite 800, Chicago, IL 60611-3215 (E-mail: dbm@prchfe.org).

[Haworth co-indexing entry note]: "But What Are We Trying to Prove?" McCurdy, David B. Co-published simultaneously in *Journal of Health Care Chaplaincy* (The Haworth Pastoral Press, an imprint of The Haworth Press, Inc.) Vol. 12, No. 1/2, 2002, pp. 151-163; and: *Professional Chaplaincy and Clinical Pastoral Education Should Become More Scientific: Yes and No* (ed: Larry VandeCreek) The Haworth Pastoral Press, an imprint of The Haworth Press, Inc., 2003, pp. 151-163. Single or multiple copies of this article are available for a fee from The Haworth Document Delivery Service [1-800-HAWORTH, 9:00 a.m. - 5:00 p.m. (EST). E-mail address: docdelivery@haworthpress.com].

10.1300/J080v12n01_17

KEYWORDS. Chaplaincy, clinical pastoral education, pastoral care, science, research

"Should professional chaplaincy and Clinical Pastoral Education (CPE) become more scientific in response to health care reform?" The question is complex, to say the least. It begs for serious exegesis, not a precipitous answer. Even so, I will lay my cards on the table at the outset. Yes, chaplaincy and CPE ought to be more "scientific," provided we tease out possible meanings of that term. This imperative should not be viewed as a response to "health care reform," for reasons I shall explain. The mischievous concluding phrase of this question–its ostensible rationale–is nonetheless the hidden key to the question itself. For, in the end, what matters is why chaplaincy and CPE should become "more scientific." I will propose that the answer lies in making the right use of whatever science chaplains and pastoral educators adopt.

A MISBEGOTTEN NOTION OF HEALTH CARE REFORM

A central premise of the question is that there actually has been, and continues to be, such a thing as "health care reform." This misapprehension may, ironically, have its genesis in the debate over the Clinton administration's comprehensive health care reform plan of 1993-94. That plan proposed a system of "managed competition" to provide universal health coverage, and thus ensure adequate access to health services for all Americans, while also controlling the costs of care. During the debate, many people associated with the healthcare industry (including not a few health care professionals) claimed that the market itself was already "reforming" health care, and was doing so quite effectively without government intrusion. Largely through the mechanisms of managed care, they contended, the market was driving down costs (or at least restraining them) and increasing efficiency. Many said–and some truly believed–that managed care would also improve the quality of care through better integration and through concerted efforts to collect clinical data and use them to develop best-practice standards of care. And the market was the engine that would bring all this to pass, in fact was already doing so.

What was forgotten in this sanguine picture of benign–even beneficent–"reform" fueled by the market was the vision of universal access based on universal coverage that lay behind the ill-fated Clinton plan. In that plan "reform" was driven by an explicit vision of justice and human good–a moral vision–that was absent from the market-driven reconfiguration of health care (O'Connell, 1994). Undoubtedly, the market has wrought enormous change, even a revolution, in healthcare delivery, and these changes have significantly affected the provision of pastoral care and education (VandeCreek, 2000a; Terrell, 2000). But to call such change "reform" is to conflate reorganization as structural re-formation with reformation as a moral enterprise. Whatever the stated reasons for the changes imposed by the market, in real time they have, for the most part, been driven by financial considerations. The *de facto* values driving this change have primarily been increasing efficiency and saving money–typically in the service of making money. Some exemplary instances of improved quality in care delivery have emerged, but they have been noteworthy precisely as exceptions.

Thus it is a disservice both to chaplains and to any future possibility of true reform to intimate that today's processes of continual restructuring and reorganization in health care amount to "reform" (VandeCreek, 2000b). On one hand, in this usage a word that normally implies a moral vision acquires negative connotations through its association with the pain of downsizing and job loss (Terrell, 2000), as if these sad and often questionable practices were an inevitable consequence of "reform." On the other hand, this misuse of the word can lend moral legitimacy to what are really market-driven pressures on chaplains and on the provision of pastoral[1] care and education.[2]

Chaplains and CPE supervisors must nonetheless acknowledge the ongoing reconfiguration of health care as an inescapable contextual reality when they reassess their ministry. It should not be the pivotal factor in their decision whether or not to become "more scientific" in their work, as I will indicate below. But neither should it–or can it–be ignored.

FIRST, THE QUESTION OF RESOURCES

The claim that the ministries of chaplaincy and CPE should be more "scientific" of course begs the question of what such a claim entails. As VandeCreek (2001b) has noted, it can be read as a claim about ministry priorities: some yet-to-be-determined "level of priority" should be given to "testing" these ministries by "scientific studies," presumably on the assumption that the results could, should, and would inform future practice.

This reading also assumes, tacitly, that adequate financial and human resources are, or can be, available to implement such a priority. I take it that it would be, first of all, a priority for the pastoral care and education *fields* as disciplines and for their professional organizations, as indeed has occurred through the COMISS initiatives and links with the National Institute for Health Care Research. At the institutional level, larger chaplaincy and education programs, programs in large health care organizations, or those affiliated with academic institutions might have an easier time embracing such a priority than programs in smaller institutions–although we should not underestimate the ingenuity of individuals and programs in "small shops." For example, chaplains in one-person departments might find experienced researchers in other disciplines with whom to collaborate (Fitchett, 1999), or smaller programs in several institutions might band together to conduct research that is centrally coordinated in some fashion.

The question of resource availability is not only important but unavoidable. At the same time, I wonder if it sometimes masks the prior question of chaplains' interest in and commitment to research. In other words, is there sufficient individual and programmatic resolve to conduct studies that chaplains and pastoral educators believe are truly worth doing? When the answer to that question is yes, my hunch is that chaplains and CPE supervisors, a resilient and resourceful group of professionals, will usually find a way to make the research happen.

THE MEANINGS OF "SCIENCE" IN THESE MINISTRIES

But what does it mean to be "scientific" in the specialized ministries of chaplaincy and CPE in the health care setting? The question can be answered from different perspectives. The discussion of adequate resources to conduct scientific studies implicitly assumes one perspective: the widely accepted understanding that science involves quantitative and/or qualitative research. In the last decade quantitative research has come to the fore in areas of interest to chaplains, as in the numerous studies exploring possible connections between spiritual or religious attitudes and practices, on one hand, and health and healing (broadly understood), on the other (Sloan et al., 2000; Cohen et al., 2000). Chaplains have participated in some of this research, and over the years they have also conducted studies specifically addressing questions within the pastoral care field. Qualitative research, taking various forms, has also emerged more prominently in the field in recent years (O'Connor et al., 2001).

Nonetheless, if a baseline for the more in "more scientific" is needed, the number of studies, both quantitative and qualitative, published in pastoral care and counseling journals has been relatively small–each kind of research comprising about five percent of the total number of articles, according to reviews of that literature conducted in 1990 (quantitative studies = 5.3% [Gartner et al.]) and 2001 (qualitative studies = 5.4% [O'Connor et al.]). It can be argued that these modest percentages provide not only an index of the commitment to "science" in chaplaincy and CPE, but also a baseline for assessing any future growth in that commitment. In any case, I believe it is worth reiterating–and emphasizing–that it is not only quantitative research that counts as "science." Numerous fields outside pastoral care and theology acknowledge the validity of qualitative research (O'Connor et al., 2001). The availability of varied qualitative methodologies both increases the potential versatility of chaplains as researchers and opens to them modalities of research that play to their existing strengths: abilities to develop relationships, listen well to people, observe the nonverbal alongside the verbal, etc., (Greiner and Bendiksen, 1994, cited in Trothen, 2001).

As to the question of fitting areas for research within this perspective on science in ministry, some areas of perennial interest come to mind. Research that helps chaplains understand the ways that patients, clinical staff members, and administrators perceive or respond to the care chaplains provide (or assess the effects of pastoral education on that care), or that helps these constituencies articulate what they see as the needs (their own or others') for pastoral care, are surely one broad area for study. "Patient satisfaction" or other "consumers'" satisfaction with pastoral care or education is one, but by no means the only, possible focus for investigation in this area. Research that seeks to identify the health-related effects of chaplains' relationships and activities with patients, thus tying those activities to the broader studies exploring the relation of religious participation or spiritual activities to health and healing, would seem another obvious candidate, although the challenge of appropriately designing such studies is by no means a small one. Studies tracing the apparent effects of identifying and intervening with patients believed to be at "spiritual risk" would be one focus in this broad area (Fitchett, 1999). Yet a third area might be studies of the possible impact of various approaches to staffing in pastoral care programs, such as further benchmark studies of staffing ratios (VandeCreek et al., 2001a), studies of the response that pastoral care volunteers or chaplains in training receive, and the like. These suggestions are but some examples.

Another, perhaps more intriguing perspective on what it means to be scientific is the range of impressions that chaplains and CPE supervisors have of what a scientific approach to their ministry would be like. In the absence (to my knowledge) of a phenomenological survey of such impressions, I will venture my own impressions of chaplains' impressions. First, it is clear that not all chaplains construe "science" in the same way. Many, I know, will have a sense that being scientific in ministry means taking seriously the kinds of qualitative and quantitative approaches and studies described above, reconsidering and revising ministry in accord with solid research findings reported in the literature, and perhaps undertaking some form of research in their own programs and practice.

For other chaplains, as in the statement from Chaplain No earlier in this volume, the perceived reality of science lies in its fixation on "numbers." In that understanding, a focus on numbers is irrelevant at best, and more likely to be hazardous to the health of pastoral care programs and the jobs of practitioners. Perhaps it conjures up the "bean counters" believed by some to inhabit health care organizations' finance offices and administrations, and thus smacks of statistics that, when reviewed, are invariably used to denigrate the importance of chaplains' ministry, and ultimately to diminish the numbers of chaplains themselves and even eliminate their programs. It is perhaps no accident that the author of that piece explicitly links "science and its methods" with "corporate values"–code, perhaps, for the priority of the bottom line–and insinuates that to engage pastoral care scientifically is simultaneously to be captured by the corporate values that have co-opted science. (Many clinicians practicing scientific medicine would, I think, take strong exception to this alleged association. In their eyes, corporate values are more likely to undermine the good that the scientific method would do were it not impeded by the "bean counters'" narrowness of vision!)

Other chaplains, I imagine, may also view "science" as a kind of numbers game but associate it, less malignantly, with the still tedious burden of keeping administratively requested statistics, perhaps without a clearly stated purpose. Still others may associate a scientific approach only with quantitative studies, without realizing that qualitative research has achieved its own legitimacy (Stannard, 2000). This admittedly impressionistic list is only a sampling. I suspect its possible value may lie in what chaplains' perceptions suggest about why some fear and/or resist the intrusion of science, as they understand it, into their ministry.

FEARS AND RESISTANCE

Some of the perceptions just mentioned lead to fears about the implications of importing "science" into chaplaincy and pastoral education, and fear may in turn lead to resistance to science so understood. One fear of chaplaincy-by-the-numbers or statistics is a fear of reductionism, such as the fear that pastoral care will be judged as if it were nothing more than those outcomes or discrete processes that researchers can measure. Such measurements may then be used, or misused, to establish performance standards, outcome goals, or staffing benchmarks that reflect a misunderstanding of what pastoral care really is.

Related fears have to do with the perceived potential of a research model to distort the very nature of pastoral care itself. I have heard it said that the invasion of pastoral care by research-based models will impose an artificial order, discipline, and structure on a field that relies on intuition, finely attuned responsiveness in the moment, and the leading of the Spirit (Kallaos, 1998, cited in Fitchett, 1999). Moreover, insofar as pressures to base pastoral practice on scientifically or statistically supported outcome studies emanate from those who wield organizational power–the authority to disburse funds and to continue, reduce, or eliminate positions and programs–survival concerns may come to dominate chaplains' participation in scientific studies and statistical assessments. Chaplains concerned with programmatic survival may spend inordinate amounts of time conducting studies that divert them from patients who should have a prior claim on their attention. (And, as chaplains already lament when administrative demands multiply, isn't availability to the patient the overriding *raison d'etre* for chaplains' institutional presence in the first place?) Survival concerns may also, it is feared, lead chaplains to use the results of studies to market or "sell" themselves (Madison, 1998) to those who have power over them and their programs. Or perhaps chaplains will seek to win greater professional or academic respectability by conforming their assessments of their work to the scientific models of those whose approval or colleagueship they seek. In either case, in their efforts to please or persuade, chaplains may betray their religious and prophetic calling (Keese, 2001) or otherwise undermine their integrity and the integrity of ministry itself (Madison, 1998).

Fears for survival, in other words, are themselves a source of fear because of their power to drive survival-oriented behavior that some chaplains question. Do not such fears lead chaplains to seek to justify their professional and programmatic existence, to try as best they can to "prove" themselves and their programs? Will fear also drive chaplains to use scientific methods, not because they "believe in" science but because ministry by the numbers may provide a last desperate hope of salvation by demonstrable works? If such motivations might lead some to science, distrust of those same motivations may lead others to turn away from a demonized science lest they become its prey. Any argument advocating scientific approaches in pastoral care and education must recognize this conflict and take it seriously, for the fears are real and chaplains know that the stakes are high. They may feel that both their survival and their integrity are at stake, and no one wants to feel forced to choose between the two. The reality of this conflict and these fears suggests the need for a further step: identifying appropriate motivations for adopting a scientific approach, and articulating the ends that it can appropriately serve.

WHAT ENDS–AND WHOSE–SHALL CHAPLAINS SERVE?

Chaplains have been urged to become more scientific in their ministries for many reasons, several of which have been alluded to in the preceding discussion. The "red thread" of a number of these considerations is programmatic survival or, where survival is not an issue–at least for now–"selling" the right parties on providing the resources necessary to maintain an already vital program or support new initiatives. Many chaplains are both weary and leery of calls to adopt new attitudes and practices in order to market pastoral care and education. When it comes to using research to "prove" the value of what they do, some bristle at the perceived enormity, futility, or hypocrisy of the task. They object that undertaking research is too daunting a project to those unskilled in research (Fitchett, 1999), it cannot in any case demonstrate the "effectiveness" of a ministry that cannot really be measured, or it is ultimately an attempt to "market" that which is not a consumer product (Keese, 2001).

I want to suggest that, on this count, the nays have it, although not necessarily for the reasons the naysayers articulate. If the aim of adopting "scientific" methods in ministry is to demonstrate to others in authority the value or validity of chaplains' ministry, and thus obtain support for programmatic survival, maintenance, or enhancement, I am not convinced that, in most instances, this approach will succeed in its aim. The reasons have much to do with the inherent limitations of research. Good research takes time–not only the day-by-day time of those who conduct it, but "longitudinal" time. It takes time to design a project;

conducting it may require months and even years; and analyzing and interpreting the results can be surprisingly time consuming. Further, sound research must have a sufficiently narrow focus in order to be manageable and to permit researchers, so far as possible, to screen out undesired variables. Finally, even the best research is, by itself, unlikely to "prove" (or disprove) its hypotheses. Results may suggest correlations without being conclusive, and correlations do not in themselves demonstrate cause and effect. Moreover, not all observers of identical study data draw the same conclusions from it; they may, for example, display differing thresholds of credulity (Stannard, 2000). And this is not even to mention the possibility that quite different results may have been obtained elsewhere in studies of similar phenomena, or the fact that not all studies are equally well conducted (Dossey, 2000). Progress in scientifically based understanding and in agreement on cause-and-effect claims proceeds slowly, and often only the cumulative impact of many studies eventually carries the persuasive day (Stannard, 2000).

Meanwhile, in the day-to-day workings of health care delivery and health care organizations, decisions about the use of resources are often made rapidly in response to circumstances and pressures that boards and administrators perceive at the time. Undertaking new research projects for the sake of programmatic survival when the pressures on resources are already acute may be a lost cause from the outset, because time simply will not allow the results to emerge and have the desired impact on decision-making. In addition, the circumscribed focus of a given study may mean that the results obtained do not provide the right kind of data, or enough of it, to influence real-time decision-making. "Too little, too late" may turn out to be all too true in many instances. On the other hand, it might be argued that administrators can be influenced favorably by the very fact that chaplains are using research methods and thus joining other clinicians and quality improvement departments in seeking to improve practice and increase efficiency. Some administrators may be less concerned about the details or validity of the research than the tangible fact that it is at least being conducted. From this perspective, undertaking research has significance as a gesture that demonstrates chaplains' professionalism, paralleling that of other clinical professionals.

Nevertheless, efforts to employ research studies for short-term or quick-fix survival purposes seem likely to yield mixed results, at best. It seems to me that the primary answer to the question, "Why be 'scientific'?" is, "We (chaplains and pastoral educators) should be more scientific so that we can learn whatever we can in order to improve our pastoral and educational practice over the long haul and, in the process, better understand our identity and the purpose of our ministry." This answer to the "Why" question is also an answer to the question, "For whose sake?" That is, chaplains need to undertake this approach for the sake of programmatic, professional, and personal enhancement and growth–which of course also means doing so for the pastoral sake of patients, families, staff, and, yes, administrators and "bean counters," too.

In this process the focus motivating a scientific approach shifts from the question, "What do we have to prove?" to "What do we hope to learn?" Marketing opportunities, programmatic survival, and even program expansion may be among the outcomes of such efforts; if they are, it is as an indirect result (however welcome), not a primary focus. The calling of chaplains begins with a call to provide ministry where it is needed and appropriate, and to do so in the best ways they know or can devise. Any approach, including research, that has potential to increase knowledge and enhance practice in this regard is surely to be sought and utilized, not treated as the enemy. As for survival, perhaps chaplains will have to live by faith that a scientific approach is worthwhile even if research is not the likely savior of programs, jobs, or respectability, but one aid (among others) to knowledge and practice. Such an attitude toward the use of scientific methods, quantitative or qualitative or both, may have the added virtue of preserving for chaplains a sense of integrity (Madison, 1998) about adopting a scientific approach. If research is not tied directly or primarily to sales, marketing, or survival concerns, some chaplains may find themselves able to undertake it with a better conscience, and thus more willingly.

SOME HOPEFUL CAUTIONS AND A SHORT WISH LIST

While it is likely that the use of various research methods will, over time, bear fruit in the form of increased understanding, I think there is a further need for sober realism. Research can be immensely engaging–or largely unexciting. Some studies reveal little that is truly new or interesting. Others may seem "off point" in relation to what health care ministry is "really" about. In short, the adoption of a scientific research focus requires patience; the fruit seldom matures quickly. But chaplains can have faith that, with time, whether in a given institution or program, or in the fields of pastoral care and education as a whole, the fruit will come.

Moreover, simply by looking through a different lens at what they do, chaplains may find that they are opened to insights that extend beyond the particular focus of a given study. More disciplined observation of the human condition, the responses that their presence and behavior elicit, and their own responses to people and their plight, may stir chaplains to see the aims and purposes of their pastoral activities, even their very identity as pastors and educators, in a new light.

In this vein, the linguistic shift from "pastoral" to "spiritual" care, embraced by both chaplaincy and CPE organizations (Anderson, 2001), seems to intimate–if not require–some kind of corresponding shift in both practice and identity. Can a scientific approach, in the form of appropriate studies, help chaplains tease out potential or real-time personal, professional, and programmatic meanings reflected in this change in language? In his recent editorial about this shift, Herbert Anderson asks several questions that might suggest areas for investigation, perhaps in particular how to "understand the ministry of chaplaincy with people who . . . identify themselves as spiritual but not religious" (2001, p. 236). Obviously, no single project can explore all the possible ramifications of the change in terminology, but perhaps a series of carefully designed, clearly focused projects could begin to sketch a picture of the practical reality accompanying the change–to help chaplains see whether and how the new "word" is becoming flesh.

For all the attention that the essays in this collection are giving to a scientific approach to ministry, I doubt that anyone engaged in pastoral care and education would deny that ministry in health care, as in other contexts, is also an art. Nor is there any need to be self-conscious about this designation or apologize for it. Even physicians who base their practice on the best science and proclaim the virtues of evidence-based medicine seldom abandon all references to medicine as an art. Indeed, "only a small minority of medical and surgical treatments have been subjected either to rigorous, controlled studies . . . or to effectiveness research" (Sharpe and Faden, 1996). Most established practices have gained their credibility through many physicians' observations of their effects on a variety of patients, and physicians know well that a standard treatment often needs to be tailored to the uniqueness of the individual patient. Observing a physician who is adept in this aspect of medical practice suggests the image of an artist at work. Chaplains, of course, have long been aware of the "art" required for ministry in health care (Cabot and Dicks, 1936). Now they are beginning to learn of the science of ministry as well. Perhaps, over time, they will learn to experience their practice as a dual yet integrated whole, as both art and science, science and art.

NOTES

1. In this paper I have chosen to use "pastoral" rather than "spiritual" to describe the care provided by chaplains, probably as much because it is the habit I developed during my years of direct involvement in chaplaincy and supervision as for any better reason. Herbert Anderson's editorial ruminations on the subject (2001) should, I hope, help spawn further reflection and discussion on the meaning of a momentous linguistic shift that deserves more scrutiny than it seems so far to have received.

2. The question posed at the outset is bifocal, encompassing both pastoral care and clinical pastoral education. In this essay I often use "chaplaincy" or "pastoral care" as an umbrella term, in part to avoid excessive repetition and cumbersome references to both pastoral care and clinical pastoral education, and in part because a "scientific" understanding of and approach to CPE would, presumably, often draw on research done by chaplains and/or research about pastoral care in the health care setting.

REFERENCES

Anderson, H. (2001). Spiritual Care: The Power of an Adjective. *Journal of Pastoral Care* 55(2) 233-237.

Cabot, R., and Dicks, R. (1926). *The Art of Ministering to the Sick.* New York: Macmillan.

Cohen, C. B. et al. (2000). Prayer as Therapy: A Challenge to Both Religious Belief and Professional Ethics. *Hastings Center Report* 30(3) 40-47.

Dossey, L. (2000). Blindsided: Criticism of CAM from an Unexpected Source. *Alternative Therapies* 6(5) 82-85.

Fitchett, G. (1999). Screening for Spiritual Risk. *Chaplaincy Today* 15(1) 2-12.

Gartner, J., Larson, D., and Vachar-Mayberry, C. (1990). A Systematic Review of the Quantity and Quality of Empirical Research Published in Four Pastoral Counseling Journals. *Journal of Pastoral Care* 55(2) 115-123.

Greiner, L. B., and Bendiksen, R. (1994). Conceptual Learning in Clinical Pastoral Education Supervisory Training: A Focus-Group Research Project with Recommendations. *Journal of Pastoral Care* 48(3) 245-256.

Kallaos, T. (1998). Agents of Healing Glad to Do More. *News Leader* [Springfield, MO], p. 7. April 19.

Keese, P. (2001). Brief Communication. *Journal of Pastoral Care* 55(3) 327-328.

Madison, T. E. (1998). Can Chaplaincy Be Sold Without Selling Out? *Chaplaincy Today* 14(2) 3-8.

O'Connell, L. J. (1994). Presentation (untitled). EHS Health Care Board of Directors retreat, Chicago, Illinois. February 5.

O'Connor, T. St. J. et al. (2001). Quantity and Rigor of Qualitative Research in Four Pastoral Counseling Journals. *Journal of Pastoral Care* 55(3) 271-280.

Sharpe, V. A., and Faden, A. I. (1996). Appropriateness in Patient Care: A New Conceptual Framework. *Milbank Quarterly* 74(1) 115-138.

Sloan, R. P. et al. (2000). Should Physicians Prescribe Religious Activities? *New England Journal of Medicine* 342(25) 1913-1916.

Stannard, R. (2000). The Prayer Experiment: Does Prayer Work? *Second Opinion* (2) 26-37.

Terrell, C. B. (2000). My Experience with Health Care Reform. In VandeCreek, L. (Ed.), *Professional Chaplaincy: What Is Happening to It During Health Care Reform?* (pp. 1-6). Binghamton, N.Y.: The Haworth Press, Inc.

Trothen, T. J. (2001). Canadian Supervised Pastoral Education–Affirmations and Ethical Queries Emerging from a Two-Year Study. *Journal of Pastoral Care* 55(4) 365-377.

VandeCreek, L. (Ed.). (2000a). *Professional Chaplaincy: What Is Happening to It During Health Care Reform?* Binghamton, N.Y.: The Haworth Press, Inc.

VandeCreek, L. (2000b). Preface. In VandeCreek, L. (Ed.), *Professional Chaplaincy: What Is Happening to It During Health Care Reform?* (pp. xi-xv). Binghamton, N.Y.: The Haworth Press, Inc.

VandeCreek, L. et al. (2001a). How Many Chaplains *Per* 100 Inpatients? Benchmarks of Health Care Chaplaincy Departments. *Journal of Pastoral Care* 55(3) 289-301.

VandeCreek, L. (2001b). Preface. *Journal of Health Care Chaplaincy* 10(1) xi-xv.

She Said, "Some Patient Needs Get Dropped Due to More Pressing Issues"

Dick Millspaugh, MDiv, BCC

SUMMARY. The engagement of the social sciences by pastoral care and education will not turn chaplains or supervisors into social scientists. Ministry is not a higher calling than science; nor will chaplains be co-oped into doing ministry by the numbers. Scientific research in pastoral care and teaching could focus on these broad areas, but administrators face multiple pressures and will not easily be convinced by rational argument. As religion and science dare to engage a meaningful dialogue; a deeper, transcendent reality will unfold. *[Article copies available for a fee from The Haworth Document Delivery Service: 1-800-HAWORTH. E-mail address: <docdelivery@haworthpress.com> Website: <http://www.HaworthPress.com> © 2002 by The Haworth Press, Inc. All rights reserved.]*

KEYWORDS. Spirituality, chaplaincy, research, science

Recently a community hospital President and Senior Executive Officer stated that patients' spiritual requests sometimes have to

---

Dick Millspaugh is President, Association of Professional Chaplains 2000-2002, Director, Chaplaincy Services, Boone Hospital Center, Columbia, MO (E-mail: dmillspa@bjc.org).

[Haworth co-indexing entry note]: "She Said, "Some Patient Needs Get Dropped Due to More Pressing Issues." Millspaugh, Dick. Co-published simultaneously in *Journal of Health Care Chaplaincy* (The Haworth Pastoral Press, an imprint of The Haworth Press, Inc.) Vol. 13, No. 1, 2002, pp. 165-170; and: *Professional Chaplaincy and Clinical Pastoral Education Should Become More Scientific: Yes and No* (ed: Larry VandeCreek) The Haworth Pastoral Press, an imprint of The Haworth Press, Inc., 2003, pp. 165-170. Single or multiple copies of this article are available for a fee from The Haworth Document Delivery Service [1-800-HAWORTH, 9:00 a.m. - 5:00 p.m. (EST). E-mail address: docdelivery@haworthpress.com].

http://www.haworthpress.com/store/product.asp?sku=J080
© 2002 by The Haworth Press, Inc. All rights reserved.
10.1300/J080v13n01_01

take second place to more pressing needs. Her statement concerned me because on a previous, more public, occasion I had heard her say that employees at her institution were empowered to do whatever it took to meet any "customer " need. When I was bold enough to ask about this apparent discrepancy, this President and SEO spoke forthrightly. "One can be idealistic, but as for me, I am realistic. I know that the nurse is the bridge between the patient and most other services. She can only do so much. Some patient needs get dropped due to more pressing issues."

In an ideal world the value of pastoral education and pastoral care would be self-evident. In an ideal world service industries would be begging to be clinical pastoral education centers. They also would be hiring professional chaplains to provide spiritual care to their employees, and perhaps to their "customers." This is not an ideal world.

My belief is that those who would argue against scientific exploration of the benefits of clinical pastoral education and chaplaincy have based their argument on several fallacies. First, to use scientific disciplines to examine pastoral care will not, as is claimed, make the art of pastoral care become a scientific discipline. One needs only to examine the close relationship of the pastoral care movement to social work, psychology and systems theory to recognize that spiritual care providers have not become social workers or psychologists. The disciplines of pastoral care and education have been deeply enriched by insights and research coming out of various professions. While the integration of basic concepts of these professions has increased the respect pastoral care educators and providers receive in the multi-disciplinary setting, the deeper value is that the teaching and provision of pastoral care has been profoundly strengthened to the benefit of those being taught and those receiving care. Such concepts as family systems, projection, introjection, personality development, and the cultural impact on perception are only a few of the multitude of concepts that now inform the delivery of pastoral care and teaching by those who are still chaplains and CPE supervisors.

The pastoral care and teaching disciplines have also been challenged to new understandings as they have been willing to engage the disciplines of both the social and physical sciences. The creation of moral and faith development models are two examples of a deepening understanding of the human condition that have brought tremendous benefit to the practice and teaching of pastoral care.

Secondly, in my opinion, it is presumptuous to believe that clinical pastoral education and chaplaincy "have a more significant calling than to be scientific." I would agree that it is a different calling, but who is to say that God is not just as involved in science as in ministry? How much love has filled the hearts of those who put themselves in harm's way to work with deadly viruses, or explore the jungles for new drugs? To idealize ministry as a more worthy calling is unseemly for a discipline that encourages its practitioners to look for a God who speaks to them in those they serve. Furthermore, such unconscious grandiosity surely isolates pastoral care and teaching from those who have much to teach us in professional ministry.

Third, to state that to engage scientific exploration of pastoral care and teaching is "trying to reduce ministry to numbers" is a specious argument. Unpublished research at Boone Hospital Center has demonstrated that patient satisfaction increases with increased chaplains' visits, and that patients are less satisfied with the chaplains' visits the longer they are hospitalized. This information informs the practice of pastoral care and teaching more than numerically. Pastoral care givers utilize the numbers to practice ministry in ways that will make more effective use of the limited amount of time, energy and resources available.

To oversimplify, one might suggest that scientific research germaine to pastoral care and education could be grouped in broad categories as follows.

- Research that is patient-results oriented, intended to inform the provision of pastoral care and education. Such research may examine how and if religious and/or spiritual ideation and/or practice may impact:
    - the patient's ability to prevent illness and/or accidents.
    - the patient's ability to cope with illness and/or accidents.
    - negative patient outcomes (morbidity, length of stay, depression, costs).
- Research that is oriented toward enlightening and strengthening the practice of pastoral care and education.

For example, focus on education theory and practice that:

- demonstrates increased learning over shorter periods of time with less resistance.
- results in empowering the patient's ability to prevent, cope with, recover from and find life giving meaning in the face of illness or accidents.

- Research that is provider-results oriented, intending to demonstrate the value of pastoral care and education to those in positions to advocate for such services. Research foci could include:
  - the intention to explore increased efficiencies, increased utilization of services, reduced costs, increased good will, all to the benefit of the provider, as well as the patient.
  - pastoral care and education issues that impact costs, increased revenue, choice of service, increased efficiencies, and other issues of importance to the value system of the provider.
  - pastoral care and education as they impact issues important to those whose opinion and influence is of critical importance to providers.

As this article specifically addresses healthcare reform, the category immediately above is most relevant to our discussion, while the first two categories may be just as important over time.

Those who argue for the need to utilize science to demonstrate the value of pastoral care and education should be both encouraged and cautioned. They should be encouraged because pastoral care and education does provide direct benefits both to the provider and to their patients, residents, clients, family, staff, and physicians. Documentation of these benefits will increase the likelihood of those benefits accruing to these populations, and secondarily to the increased access of pastoral care and education service providers to these persons.

On the other hand, those seeking to scientifically demonstrate the value of pastoral care and education to providers should be cautioned. Those who determine if pastoral care and education services will exist in provider institutions are influenced by a myriad of powerful forces. To assume that these providers will be easily persuaded by rational scientific documentation of the value of pastoral care and education to their institutions, their clientele and staff would be naive.

As an example of the complexity of the influences bearing down upon a provider consider the following assumptions. The provider will probably be more influenced by the factors listed below than by rigorous scientific study.

- His or her own experience with the benefits and/or liabilities of religion and/or spirituality especially as mediated through his or her own family history.

- The subjective opinions of the medical staff as regards religion and/or spirituality, again, often mediated through their own historical experience.
- The perceived economic environment within the institution and the industry.
- The culture of the institution and the locale.
- The requirements of regulatory agencies.
- The interpretation of the separation of church and state clause.

To be realistic, pastoral care givers and teachers compete for limited resources. Health care reform is driven by this reality combined with the ideal of seeking to provide more efficacious health care. Therefore pastoral care givers and teachers would be cautioned to be as "wise as serpents and as gentle as doves." Wisdom in this case means to recognize that pastoral care givers and teachers will have to speak the language of the foreign land in which they reside if they hope to be given a home. That language is science and economics, neither of which are the native tongue of the pastoral care provider or teacher. To learn to speak this second and third language, however, does not mean that the chaplain or CPE supervisor has to give up his or her native language–the theology that grounds the provision of and the teaching of pastoral care.

As those who critique the use of science in examining pastoral care and teaching quickly point out, there is an inherent danger that in speaking a second language one may forget one's mother tongue. However, professional associations, journals, and colleagues can help one stay grounded in the practice of ministry, even while in the foreign land.

I believe this is not an "either/or" issue but rather a "both/and" issue. In my opinion, science explores "facts" available through the senses in a way that seeks to demonstrate and then replicate the truth of a specific hypothesis. Religion, on the other hand, seeks to provide ritual, creeds, beliefs, practices, and symbols to help persons make a connection to the transcendent and to foster healthy community. Religion and theology also seek to demonstrate and then replicate the truth as found by experience, reason, tradition and revelation.

Both science and religion operate as agencies of faith. Science maintains the faith that reality can be discerned through the senses and is replicable. Religion maintains that reality is larger than that which can be discerned through the senses and is both knowable and unknowable.

So I would propose that we are about a "both/and" issue. Reality, in my opinion, is finally larger than either religion or science can discern or define. So we need both religion and science to inform our practice of pastoral care and teaching. There is a larger reality beyond either science or religion. We should encourage those who wish to explore truth in science and those who wish to explore truth in religion to join forces to discover the Truth beyond.

Those who fear that scientific research will co-opt the pastoral care and education enterprise may have unwittingly fallen into promoting a world view that has separated reality into fragments. In pre-critical thought the spirit and material world were one. The age of reason birthed critical thinking and gave rise to the scientific method. While many benefits have poured forth from this worldview, it also divided religion and science in two. To advocate staying outside the world of science is to continue to support such a divided worldview.

I argue that a post-critical world view will unfold in our distant future. In this world a truth more inclusive than religion and science will be birthed. In this new view a deeper sense of the oneness of what we now call the material and the spiritual will emerge in a way that rings true to the depths of who we are and what the universe is. This unfolding will happen precisely through the engagement and dialogue of science and religion, resulting not in one discipline subsuming the other, but in an entirely new understanding, richer, more profound and more revealing of the divine than either current states of religion or science.

In order to foster this dialogue science will need to own that the scientific method is a belief statement in and of itself, and give tolerance to a view that there may be realities that cannot be measured, that realities may exist both within and beyond time and space. On the other hand religion will need to come to honor the possibility that the Holy may reveal truth in the scientific endeavor.

The hospital administrator was correct in saying, "Some patient needs get dropped due to more pressing issues." Resources and time are limited. Ideally health care reform would highlight the value of and fund the provision of spiritual care and teaching. This may not happen. Therefore, it is imperative that chaplains, supervisors and their associations and faith communities engage in dialogue with science and research as one means, but only as one means, to see that the spiritual needs and education of those we serve are not dropped.

Respecting the Dual Sided Identity of Clinical Pastoral Education and Professional Chaplaincy: The Phenomenological Research Model

Marie-Line Morin, PhD

SUMMARY. The question discussed in this volume opens a debate on what kind of scientific research model should be used by professional chaplaincy and Clinical Pastoral Education (CPE). The problem begins with the assumption that "becoming more scientific" means using the natural sciences approach employed by psychology; an approach unsuitable to account for factors relative to faith, spiritual and religious issues. I argue that CPE and professional chaplaincy need to be more scientific but not necessarily under the natural sciences model. Considering the predominance of that model in psychology, I believe pastors and chaplains should resist pressures to rely on the natural science model and adopt instead models that respect their dual sided identity. I conclude by suggesting that the phenomenological research model best allows investigation of patients' spiritual as well as psychological issues.

Marie-Line Morin is on the Faculty of Theology, Ethics and Philosophy, University of Sherbrooke, Sherbrooke, Quebec, J1L 2N3, Canada (E-mail: mimorin@courrier.usherb.ca).

[Haworth co-indexing entry note]: "Respecting the Dual Sided Identity of Clinical Pastoral Education and Professional Chaplaincy: The Phenomenological Research Model." Morin, Marie-Line. Co-published simultaneously in *Journal of Health Care Chaplaincy* (The Haworth Pastoral Press, an imprint of The Haworth Press, Inc.) Vol. 13, No. 1, 2002, pp. 171-183; and: *Professional Chaplaincy and Clinical Pastoral Education Should Become More Scientific: Yes and No* (ed: Larry VandeCreek) The Haworth Pastoral Press, an imprint of The Haworth Press, Inc., 2003, pp. 171-183. Single or multiple copies of this article are available for a fee from The Haworth Document Delivery Service [1-800-HAWORTH, 9:00 a.m. - 5:00 p.m. (EST). E-mail address: docdelivery@haworthpress.com].

10.1300/J080v13n01_02

KEYWORDS. Chaplaincy, spirituality, science, research

Clinical Pastoral Education (CPE) and professional chaplaincy focus on issues related to faith, spirituality, and psychological concerns such as depression and anxiety. Unlike other health professionals, this ministry addresses these issues from two different fields of expertise, the spiritual and the psychological. The question posed in the title of this volume refers inevitably to the assumptions that all professionals follow the same model of science. What this question really asks, therefore, is whether CPE and professional chaplaincy should buy into the scientific research principles of the natural sciences. The field of psychology does so, applying scientific principles from the natural sciences to the study of the human mind, behaviour, and attitudes. Because CPE and professional chaplaincy give attention to the spiritual and psychological needs of their patients, it is appropriate to ask whether they should employ the scientific methods of the natural sciences. The problem begins at that very point–the assumption that "becoming more scientific" means using the methods of the natural sciences.

Chaplain No and Chaplain Yes whose materials appear near the front of this volume have opposite arguments. The first states that CPE and professional chaplaincy have the moral obligation to resist becoming more scientific in order to preserve the essence of ministry whose first calling is to "represent the love of the Transcendent." The second argues that these professions also have the moral obligation; it is to become more scientific in order to demonstrate to peer health professionals the helpfulness of what they intuitively know to be helpful in their ministry. Although I agree with both authors on some issues, I believe the arguments of each contain problematic assumptions. It is necessary, indeed, to keep the essence of CPE and professional chaplaincy, an essence that can neither be "reduced to numbers" nor be justified by "statistically demonstrating its outcomes." It is also important that these professions not hold themselves "outside of the circle of other professionals" as if scientific methods were irrelevant to their ministry. I maintain, however, that the positions taken by Chaplain No and Chaplain Yes are troublesome because they both assume the use of the natural science model used in psychology. My stance is that CPE and professional chaplaincy need to be scientific but not necessarily in the same way as the natural sciences. Pastoral researchers in both domains, like other professionals who are interdisciplinary in nature, should identify and consolidate their own research principles and criteria that respect specific characteristics of their professions. In the discussion that follows, therefore, I will first discuss some of the reasons why CPE and chaplains are uneasy with science. Second, I will comment on the need for CPE and professional chaplaincy to resist social pressures to follow the current scientific research model borrowed from natural science. Third, I will suggest a model that they can use to investigate spiritual and psychological issues that is known for its scientific validity.

WHY CHAPLAINS MAY BE UNCOMFORTABLE WITH BEING SCIENTIFIC

To begin, the care offered by pastors and chaplains is based on spiritual and religious teachings such as the Christian message of faith and hope. Whatever the difficulties encountered, they will try to remind the ill that the love of the God, through Christ, is always there for them. Prayers, reading the Bible, trusting in God and helping others, become means by which distress can be alleviated. This message implies the acceptance of scriptural contents as the "Word of God" regardless of the fact that this cannot be proven scientifically through contemporary research models. Instead, its validity is rooted in the apostles' testimony about their experience of Christ's love in their life and in the testimonies from people who, till this day, continue to assert such personal experiences of Christ's love, presence and intervention in their life. The scientific basis for all this is assured by theology, also considered a science, but under a different model than the one used in psychology and the natural sciences.

Additionally, pastors and chaplains also rely on psychological knowledge to assist patients in their sufferings. When attending someone with depressive symptoms, for example, they need to be aware of psychological research results that point the way toward helpful interventions. Now, psychological research is rooted in a completely different logic than that of the spiritual or religious perspective. Indeed, research models in modern psychology are borrowed from the natural sciences and based on the following presupposition: Reality is defined in terms of that which is observable and measurable (Croteau, 1981). Results are considered valid inasmuch as they are generated from statistical methods and empirical data gathered according to operationally defined variables. The cognitive-behavioural school of thought is the best example of how this model is adapted in psychology.

The basis for the spiritual and the psychological scientific approaches is so different that a majority of professionals believe they are incompatible. From a strictly psychological viewpoint the spiritual (or religious) approach is often considered unreliable because God, revelation, and faith cannot be empirically observed or measured through operational variables. No one can, indeed, calculate statistically the effects of grace and God's intervention since these cannot be seen, heard, or felt through the senses in ways compatible with modern scientific studies. A reliable research project in which God's intervention is the independent variable and human response is the dependant variable cannot produce convincing results. From a pastoral or religious perspective, results from psychological research are often considered "dry," technical and too limited. Relying on human means alone to overcome issues that transcend human reality such as spiritual responses to the human beings' quest for meaning and purpose is likely considered reductive by pastors and chaplains. God's power and infinite manifestations cannot, indeed, be solely reduced to human understandings, even when such understandings are based on statistical calculations.

Thus, as described in Table 1, the underlying presuppositions of the spiritual and the natural science approaches are strikingly opposite.

In spite of that apparent dichotomy, clinical pastoral educators and chaplains continue to use both approaches in their ministry. They are more comfortable, however, with the spiritual/religious approach than the psychological. Since faith and spirituality are the core issues in the pastoral aspect of their ministry, persons such as Chaplain No wonder why we need scientific research results at all. If ministry is oriented towards spirituality and religion, why should research based on psychological principles be necessary? Some may even go as far as thinking that if the word of the "perfect" God is trustworthy, any information coming from "imperfect" human beings is misleading, especially when results originate from a natural science perspective that considers spiritual matters as unreal and unreliable. Such a position, however, is vulnerable to fanatical interpretations of the Bible and devastating types of interventions. The interpretation of God's Word can be so diverse and contradictory that some principles ensuring reliability of such interpretations and intervention are recommended. This alone justifies the need for some kind of scientific research in CPE and professional chaplaincy

TABLE 1. Presuppositions of Spiritual and Natural Science Research Approaches

Presuppositions In Theology*	Presuppositions In Psychology**
• God and life after death exist; thus human beings are created in the image of God and aim at returning to him; • religion is rooted in God's revelation or intervention through the prophets and apostles; • human beings are free to choose between good and bad; • peoples' lives ultimately find their meaning, purpose and harmony through communion with God; • religious experiences refer to God revealing his presence.	• God's existence and life after death are not addressed; thus human beings are biologically determined or conditioned by early childhood environment or intra-psychic organization; • religion is a father complex projection • freedom is rooted in the person's capacity to choose to be congruent to one's actualization process; • meaning and purpose in life is based on what is found by self, solely; • religious phenomena are explained by natural, human psychological disposition to peak-experiences.

*These presuppositions reflect teachings from the main Christian traditions.
**These presuppositions reflect these prominent schools of thought in psychology: cognitive-behavioral, psychoanalytic, and humanistic-existential.

and supports the claims of Chaplain Yes in favour of more science–although this position needs refinement.

Considering all this, my position regarding whether CPE and professional chaplaincy should become more scientific is the following: They need to be scientific, but also need to take account of the irreconcilable dichotomy between the spiritual/religious and the natural science approaches. In fact, to address that issue, I prefer to ask the following question: "Should CPE and professional chaplaincy be scientific under the same model as other sciences?" My answer to that question is "No!" Science in CPE and chaplaincy should be defined on the basis of respect for their unique identities, and be done in a way that allows integration of the spiritual/religious and psychological dimensions of persons who receive pastoral services.

SCIENCE AND SPIRITUALITY/RELIGION IN CONTEMPORARY SOCIETY

In the modern western world, the natural science model appears to be the most reliable source of information. Results generated through empirical research that include operationalized variables and observable data tend to be interpreted as "truths" by which people should orient their lives and make decisions. This scientific model has generated so many new discoveries in the last century that our way of approaching reality has changed radically. Our approach to life is now tinted by the various possibilities of technology allowing individual satisfaction (Taylor, 1989) where inner feelings and personal actualization have precedence over other values such as the love of neighbours. This suggests a new paradigm in comparison to past generations where life seemed to be more readily oriented toward obedience to God with concern for the well-being of neighbours and society. Spiritual and religious dimensions of life, then, seemed more intertwined with everyday events, nature, and persons, resulting in spontaneous inner movements toward faith (Vergote, 1971). One of the characteristics of modernity is that religion and faith do not tend to emerge spontaneously as part of life experience with a natural sense of awe in which people feel they are one with God the Creator. Influenced by Cartesian thought, the western world's rapport with spirituality and religion is characterized by a clear distinction between subject and object. Faith and spirituality now tend to be the result of personal choices and experiences occurring when the person is confronted with the limits of life. People turn to God when they need an answer to troublesome issues such as suffering, inner emptiness, and the search for meaning (Vergote, 1971).

When spiritual and religious matters seem to be accidental experiences, when science appears to be most reliable in predicting matters associated to a great variety of events, the natural science model easily becomes the ultimate point of reference from which to base our most important decisions in life. For example in matters referring to "cloning," little attention is given to God and spiritual consequences when considering ethical risks associated to such experimentation.

In spite of its popularity, we need to remember that this scientific method is only a product of human intelligence. The principles and criteria used to declare what we consider reliable are produced by human minds and thus limited and limitative. Science does not generate "truth," it generates "probabilities." That is to say, it creates more or less reliable results about the predictability of diverse events, variables and phenomena. The same results found reliable in one study may, therefore, be found unreliable in further research. Results demonstrate responses to certain stimulants at a certain time, under certain conditions–X dependant variables in the face of Y independent variables.

Does that mean that truth is a matter of spiritual and religious beliefs alone? Although most of the great religious traditions claim to teach the truth about God's message to human beings, the mere fact that people are divided into so many different interpretations brings doubt about such beliefs. Experience shows that the interpretation of the Bible and Christ's message is constantly subject to projection and biased personal interpretation. The history of religion shows that what is considered a fundamental theological principle of truth in one denomination is contested in another. Risks of misinterpreting the Lord's word are constantly present, no matter how intelligent, wise and mature one's faith. Such risks invite everyone to be critical about their own understanding of scripture.

Although CPE and chaplaincy may first rely on spiritual and religious approaches in ministry, they also know that interpretations of God's word are limited. That is why they usually admit that science is necessary as regards spiritual and religious issues. Admitting the importance of the science of theology, for example, also means recognizing the need for science in CPE and professional chaplaincy. Knowing the place of science in modern societies, they cannot afford to leave aside knowledge generated by the natural sciences in spite of its limitations. Once recognizing its limits, however, they need to move beyond the "trap" in which the natural science model used in psychology appears to be the only model from which science is done. In fact, recognizing the limitations in both aspects of their ministry the challenge for CPE and professional chaplaincy is to find an integrative point for the spiritual/religious and the psychological dimensions of their professional identity from which to do scientific research.

FINDING THE SCIENTIFIC INTEGRATIVE POINT FOR PSYCHOLOGICAL AND SPIRITUAL/RELIGIOUS DIMENSIONS

My comments so far raise the question of social pressure based on preferences for a particular scientific approach over another. Now, such preferences are not indicators of what is most reliable. Indeed, if we consider that each of the two approaches has its own limitations, perhaps it is useful to think that both are necessary and need to be surpassed–integrating the good in each approach and moving a step beyond. When considering the differences presented in Table 1, it may appear impossible to integrate the two. This may be true, indeed, if we look at the dilemma solely on the bases of the presuppositions and social preferences. To find an integrative point to define science in CPE and professional chaplaincy we need, first, to remember that pastoral education and chaplaincy are oriented toward persons experiencing both psychological and spiritual or religious sufferings simultaneously. Questions such as "Why am I suffering?" "Is God present in this loss?" "Can God give me relief?" are present along with requests such as "I need something that will alleviate my depressive symptoms," or " Help me overcome suicidal thoughts." In such situations, both the psychological and the spiritual/religious dimensions of the person are present and need to be taken in consideration as a whole. We also need to remember that human beings, in their psychological and spiritual essences can never be completely understood or accounted for through the natural science model with its statistical and probabilistic approach.

A person's subjectivity, freedom to decide, conscience, will and capacity to relate to God transcend the methodological constraints imposed by the principles and criteria guiding natural science research. They cannot be directly observed and measured. When that model is used to study humans, essential aspects of their fundamental being are left out. For example, when a subject says "I feel anxious," there is a subject, "I," experiencing anxiety. From a spiritual/religious or theological point of view, the "I" is acknowledged, with the help of philosophical reasoning, as being a central entity from which meaning and purpose is deployed (Croteau, 1981)–subjectivity, freedom, conscience, etc., emerge from the subject said to be an "I." On the contrary, when restricting our study to the natural science model, we are forced to admit with Hume, that "I" cannot be seen or felt because "when I enter most intimately into what I call myself I always stumble in some particular perception [. . .] I can never catch *myself* at any time without a perception, I can never observe anything but the perception" (as quoted in Levin, 1992). Faithful to the philosophical presupposition of observable reality, Hume is unable to conclude that perceptions he observes emerge from a subject: "I" is the one who perceives. He is forced to explain human subjectivity by the following assertion: "mankind [. . .] is nothing but a bundle or collection of different perceptions." To admit the existence of "I" as a subjective entity, as substance or substrate of experience, detaining freedom, conscience, will, and openness to God, one has to allow a space for reasoning and interpreting observed data from a different stance than that of natural science (Croteau, 1981).

To find a scientific integrative point for psychological and spiritual/religious dimensions in CPE and professional chaplaincy research, we need to do science out of a model which dares to question the prominent research model. We should not necessarily do more science in the present psychological model nor should we stay away from it in order to remain faithful to traditional religious teachings. We need to do research from a third point of view, transcending while integrating the other two. The new model must allow in-depth analysis of phenomenon from the subjective perspective of both the psychological and the spiritual or religious dimensions of persons. While different research models are available, the model I suggest below is remarkably suited for CPE and professional chaplaincy research. In the remainder of this article, I will provide a brief introduction to the phenomenological psychology model developed by A. Giorgi (1985) at Duquesne University and refined by Croteau (1994) (who thoroughly studied Giorgi's approach from a psycho-philosophical perspective and called it "existential phenomenology").

The phenomenological psychology research model is an experiential approach to the study of phenomena, rooted in phenomenology and existentialist psychology, two philosophical orientations developed in reaction to the natural science model. Without going back to philosophical idealism which modern psychology tried to evade by adopting natural science presuppositions, this approach intends to overcome the separation between subjects and object created by Cartesian philosophy underlying natural science. The basic principle underlying the phenomenological psychology model comes from Husserl, the father of phenomenology, who insisted it was necessary to "come back to the things themselves as they appear immediately to conscience before any theorization or philosophical explanation" (Croteau, 1994). In doing so, the analyses of human beings' psyche are not subject to mathematical divisions of so-called objective observable data. Instead, the subject, as a whole, is considered as data; that is to say, his intellectual and spiritual intuitions present in his experience of reality are included in the data, as much as the sensible experiences felt in the body and senses (Croteau, 1994). While Husserl's philosophy was vulnerable to charges that it was idealistic and disconnected from concrete experience, Giorgi refined it into a research model where existentialist principles are included as a way to give attention to human beings' concrete lived experiences. Thus, considering subjects' conscience of "things themselves" in their concrete experience of the world ensures researchers' access to data reflecting the global reality as it is lived by these subjects. The goal, in this approach, is to let the information used for theorizing emerge from human subjects without interfering, or at least, interfering as little as possible. Instead of starting off by identifying a hypothesis and an operational model, existential phenomenology (phenomenological psychology) starts with subjects and at-length descriptions of their experience. It aims to identify the fundamental structure of meaning and purpose experienced in any given existential phenomenon (Husserl in Giorgi, 1985). Classifying, interpreting, theorizing comes after the "things themselves" are collected "as they immediately appear to conscience."

This model allows consideration of spiritual or religious experiences such as one's faith in God, one's experience of his grace and love as well as psychological experiences like feelings, attitudes, schemas, and intra-psychic organization as they appear to subjects' conscience and as they impact one another. Indeed, a wide variety of experiences can be analyzed with this approach, as they relate to persons' spiritual/religious and psychological dimensions. Research based on this approach will give valuable scientifically based information because these fundamental structures are understood as predictable organization to a variety of phenomena. It can thus help pastoral clinicians and chaplains demonstrate to health care managers, the scientific value of their work based on data respectful of their dual sided identity. In that sense, the existential phenomenological approach constitutes a scientific model suited for CPE and professional chaplaincy from which to do research from an integrative point between the psychological and spiritual/religious dimension in human beings.

Other approaches may be helpful in finding such an integrative but phenomenological psychology has the advantage of allowing a deep understanding of various phenomenon in that perspective. To become acquainted with this model, readers can refer to A. Giorgi's work itself and other authors listed in the references. I now provide some additional details concerning the principles underlying this model.

PRINCIPLES
OF THE EXISTENTIAL PHENOMENOLOGY MODEL

The existential phenomenology model implies that human beings, closely linked to the world in which they live, experience themselves as beings-in-the-world, as having a consciousness of their own and as being free to make choices and decisions on their own account. Unlike animals and things human subjects are characterized by what Croteau (1994) calls a "consciousness-incarnate-in-the-world" and "consciousness-incarnate-intentional." The world experienced by such a consciousness-incarnate refers to three modalities: their connection to (a) the world around (physical and material things–Umwelt); (b) the world with others (people with whom one relates–Mitwelt); (c) the world within (thoughts, feelings, desires revealing how one experiences self–Eigenwelt).

These categories help the researcher clarify the variety of elements gathered from the interview with a subject. Croteau's understanding of phenomenological psychology also includes two more categories to account for the subjects' aspiration for meaning and purpose; they are (d) the will to meaning and (e) the sense of responsibility. All five categories are used to classify information gathered from interviews with subjects in such a way that researchers can identify the essence of the phenomenon–or meaning structure. This essence is then expressed in terms of meaning and purpose originating from the encounter between an aim (something for which the subject aims–noesis) and the object itself (the good, the reality, thing aimed–noema). The meaning and purpose resulting from the meeting of that which the conscience aims and the thing itself which is aim is called the "intentionnality." Intentionnalities derived from essential meaning and purpose are considered as the expression of the meaning structure faithful to the person's will of meaning in a given phenomenon.

Unlike traditional empirical psychological research, the focus of this method is not to aim at probabilities and inferences that can be generalized to larger population. Its focus is on identification of stable laws, fundamental structures and idiosyncratic profiles of invariant structure of meaning in a particular phenomenon. The meaningfulness of the type of information resulting from this approach is based on the stability of phenomenological meaning structures. Redundancy of meaning structure in repeated interview based research with people having experienced similar phenomenon is the criteria for validity; finding repetition in the essence of a given phenomenon generates meaningful understanding of that phenomenon which can by used in clinical settings as well as theoretical elucidation. Dukes (1984) gives a clear example of invariant structures of meaning in the phenomenon of loss or death of a loved one. In all cases, regardless of difference in facts surrounding such an experience, the following structure is there: (1) the initial refusal–insisting that it is not or cannot be; (2) an attempt to construct circumstances in which it (the death) need not have been–"if only" I had done this or not done that–which leads to self-blame; (3) an attempt to preserve control over the uncontrollable; (4) the shutting down of being–food has no taste, etc.; (5) the remembering of long forgotten moments. Dukes explains:

> Loss, the death of a loved one, is a universally and distinctly human experience that has an inherent logic, a rhyme and rhythm of is own, and that logic or structure is the same for any human being

who has ever suffered loss. The facts of the loss, certainly, differ from case to case [. . .]. But the experience of grief is the same [invariant structure of meaning], whether the loved one is a puppy, a parakeet or a child. (200)

Validity of this method is thus based on the invariant structures identified repeatedly in different people experiencing a similar given phenomenon.

The meaning structures are identified using two fundamental principles: the phenomenological reduction and eidetic reduction. These principles imply that the researcher adopts a neutral position, as much as possible, from any preconceived ideas, values or theoretical explanations of the interview content. The phenomenological reduction consists in putting in parentheses one's natural attitude of the mind toward reality and theoretical presuppositions about the findings–as much as one can abstract from one's own theoretical background. Once the researcher identifies his or her theoretical background, he or she chooses not to refer to it while interpreting and attempting to describe the content of the interview as it appears to the subject's consciousness-incarnate. From there, the researcher considers the experience as it is signified and understood by the person who describes it, without trying to define whether it is measurable or verifiable (Giorgi, 1985) or to make interpretations from preconceived theory. The aim is to focus on knowledge of subjects' meaning structure per se rather than to verify whether the meaning itself is true or false.

Eidetic reduction refers to the process by which the researcher allows a structure of meaning to emerge from the interview content–also called the essence of the phenomenon. In this procedure, the researcher eliminates all the unnecessary elements (accidental or secondary things) in the discourse under study and keeps the core essence or the invariable structure of meaning given by that same person in a particular psychic phenomenon.

The technique by which the researcher applies these two principles is called the "free imaginary variation" Croteau (1994) quotes Merleau-Ponty who describes this technique in the following terms:

(free imaginary variation is) to allow a concrete experience to float in one's mind so as to let oneself imagine that experience in every possible modified aspect; what remains invariable thereafter is the essence of the phenomenon under examination. (Merleau-Ponty in Croteau, 1994; unpublished; no page number)

In this process, the researcher attempts, after eliminating peripheral aspects of the person's discourse, to identify with as much accuracy as possible the "invariable contingents"–that which is constant and relevant to the subjective structure of meaning–describing that person's way of being-in-the-world in relation to a given phenomenon or experience (Giorgi, 1985).

REFERENCES

Croteau, J. (1981). L'homme: Sujet ou objet, prolémènes philosophiques à une psychologie scientifico-humaniste. Paris: Desclée.

Croteau, J. (1994). Précis de psychologie phénoménologico-existentielle, Initiation à son approche, sa méthode, à ses techniques d'analyse. Unpublished document. Deschatelet: Ottawa.

Dukes, S. (1984). Phenomenological Methodology in the Human Sciences. *Journal of Religion and Health*, 23:3. 197-203.

Giorgi, A. (1985). Phenomenology and Psychological Research, Duquesne Université Press.

Klein, P. and Westcott, M. R. (1994). The Changing Character of Phenomenological Psycholgy. *Canadian Psychology*, 35:2. 133-158.

Levin, J. D. (1992). *Theories of the Self*. Washington: Hemisphere Publishing Corporation.

Osborne, J. W. (1994). Some Similarities and Differences Among Phenomenological and Other Methods of Psychological Qualitative Research. *Canadian Psychology*, 35:2. 167-189.

Taylor, C. (1989). *Sources of the Self, The making of the Modern Identity*, Cambridge, Massachusetts: Harvard University Press.

Valle, R. S. and Halling, S. (1989). *Existential-Phenomenological Perspectives in Psychology*. New York: Plenum Press.

Vergote, A. (1971). *Psychologie religieuse*. Bruxelles: Dessart.

The Search for Truth:
The Case for Evidence Based Chaplaincy

Thomas St. James O'Connor, ThD

SUMMARY. Chaplaincy and medical science are in search of truth. Should chaplaincy become more scientific in response to health care reform? Yes is the answer. Chaplaincy ought to become more based in evidence for the following reasons. First, the health care culture is evidence based and chaplaincy needs to speak that language. Second, chaplaincy and science are not opposed. Third, tradition-driven chaplaincy already utilizes medical evidence. Fourth, spirituality is the domain of chaplaincy and other health care disciplines have provided the research in our domain. However, if chaplaincy becomes more scientific, it does not mean that chaplaincy will maintain or grow in its position in health care reform. Health care reform in relation to chaplaincy is driven more by values than evidence. *[Article copies available for a fee from The Haworth Document Delivery Service: 1-800-HAWORTH. E-mail address: <docdelivery@haworthpress.com> Website: <http://www.HaworthPress.com> © 2002 by The Haworth Press, Inc. All rights reserved.]*

Thomas St. James O'Connor is Associate Professor, Pastoral Care and Counseling, Waterloo Lutheran Seminary, Waterloo, Ontario, Canada and Associate Clinical Professor, Family Medicine, McMaster University and Senior Chaplain, Hamilton Health Sciences, Hamilton, Ontario, Canada (E-mail: toconnor@hhsc.ca).

Special thanks to Delton Glebe, ThD, and Elizabeth Meakes, MTS, for providing helpful feedback on an earlier version of this manuscript.

[Haworth co-indexing entry note]: "The Search for Truth: The Case for Evidence Based Chaplaincy." O'Connor, Thomas St. James. Co-published simultaneously in *Journal of Health Care Chaplaincy* (The Haworth Pastoral Press, an imprint of The Haworth Press, Inc.) Vol. 13, No. 1, 2002, pp. 185-194; and: *Professional Chaplaincy and Clinical Pastoral Education Should Become More Scientific: Yes and No* (ed: Larry VandeCreek) The Haworth Pastoral Press, an imprint of The Haworth Press, Inc., 2003, pp. 185-194. Single or multiple copies of this article are available for a fee from The Haworth Document Delivery Service [1-800-HAWORTH, 9:00 a.m. - 5:00 p.m. (EST). E-mail address: docdelivery@haworthpress.com].

10.1300/J080v13n01_03

KEYWORDS. Chaplaincy, religion, science, research

When I began as a chaplain at Chedoke-McMaster Hospitals in 1992, I attended a number of staff meetings to introduce myself and to explain the role of chaplaincy. At one of these meetings, a physician asked me: "What evidence does chaplaincy have to show that it can help our patients?" Spontaneously, I blurted out: "We walk by faith not by evidence!" However, the question stayed with me and sent me in search of the evidence. The environment in which I work values evidence based health care. By the time I arrived as a chaplain, almost every discipline in health sciences had adopted to some degree the evidence-based approach (Donald, 1994). Should chaplaincy become more scientific in response to health care reform? I say yes, based on four reasons.

1. THE SCIENTIFIC CULTURE IN HEALTH CARE
IS EVIDENCE BASED

The faculty of health sciences at McMaster in Hamilton, Ontario is the home of evidence-based health care. McMaster is recognized as the first place that rigorously developed the approach back in the early seventies (Rosenberg and Donald, 1995; O'Connor and Meakes, 1998). Evidence based health care is ". . . the conscientious, explicit and judicious use of current best evidence in making decisions about the care of individual patients" (Cited, McKibbon, 1999, 2). Evidence based health care is research driven.

Evidence is published research. McKibbon (1999) notes seven levels of published research in evidence-based health care. Level 1 is the discussion of ideas based on clinical experience. Here, the research is more reflective and theoretical but it is based on the clinical experience of the researcher and others. Level 2 is the use of case studies. The published research of much of the chaplaincy literature is at level 1 and 2 (O'Connor et al., 2002; Larson et al., 1990). Level three is laboratory testing. Level 4 is the evidence from testing on animals. Level 5 is the evidence from phase 1 trials on humans. Usually the sample is small and not randomly selected. Level 6 is the evidence from phase 2 of trials. Here the sample is larger and could be randomized. Level 7 is the evidence from randomized control trials (RCT). A RCT that has been replicated is the highest form of evidence–the most reliable and valid. In level 7, scientists believe that one has arrived at the truth and some consider the findings of an RCT as the highest form of knowledge (Mays and Pope, 1995).

Qualitative research is also part of evidence-based health care and Marks (1999) notes that it has become acceptable in health care research. O'Connor and Meakes (1998) place qualitative research between level 2 and level 3. Scientific then means being based in empirical evidence. Thus, in scientific evidence based health care, there are various kinds of evidence from research. There is quantitative, qualitative and case study along with ideas rooted in clinical experience. All these kinds of research evidence are not equal. The highest form of evidence is the double blind, randomized control trial. The lowest form is the ideas that stem from clinical experience.

One of the critiques of evidenced-based medicine is the poor place given to clinical wisdom that includes the doctor-patient relationship. In the schema outlined, there is no mention of clinical wisdom. The assumption might be that any evidence from levels 1-7 that contradicts a physician's clinical experience ought to override clinical experience. The *Lancet*, in an editorial (Sept. 23, 1995), critiques evidence-based medicine as elitist and negating clinical experience. Rather, the clinical experience and patient relationship are vital and sound evidence-based medicine "builds upon rather than disparages or neglects, the evidence gained from good clinical skills and sound clinical experience" (cited, p. 785). One sees here the need in health care for both science based on evidence, as well as sound clinical experience that takes seriously the dynamics of the relationship with the patient.

Health care chaplaincy exists in this culture of evidence based health care. Evidence based language and concepts are the dominant narrative. The theological-spiritual language of chaplaincy is a minor narrative. Chaplaincy must be familiar with evidence-based language and narrative and be able to speak it. Chaplains fear that if they move more towards a scientific, evidence based approach they will lose their religious traditions and the role of faith. The concern is that the scientific melting pot will erase chaplaincy's unique contribution. Is this necessarily so?

I believe that chaplaincy can be both rooted in tradition and evidence based (scientific). It is not an either/or but a both/and approach. The Canadian experience of a bilingual, bicultural nation indicates that different narratives can co-exist and co-operate without the loss of identity. Minorities can thrive, have their identities and be connected to the majority (Ignatieff, 2000). They learn from each other. Canada is not a melting pot but a cultural mosaic. Chaplaincy in developing a more scientific evidence based approach ought to keep in mind the image of a cultural mosaic.

2. RELIGION AND SCIENCE ARE NOT OPPOSED

A second argument for chaplains becoming more scientific is the belief that religion and science are not opposed. Both religion and science seek truth. Science relies on truth discovered through empirical means and religion relies on truth discovered through sacred texts and traditions. Ian Barbour (1997) notes four relationships between science and religion. One is conflicted where each seeks to prove that the other is wrong on an issue. An example is the controversy over the theory of evolution and some literal interpretations of the creation story in Genesis 1 and 2. Here, certain religious interpretations disagree with certain scientific interpretations and each strives to prove the other wrong. A second relationship emphasizes separate spheres of expertise. Religion deals with spiritual matters and science deals with material matters. In this view, these two realms co-exist and are separate similar to the separation of Church and State. The argument to not make chaplaincy scientific usually flows from this second relationship. A third relationship is that there are certain common points between religion and science. Both seek the truth and seek to understand and explain the origins of the universe. Both are concerned with physical, mental and emotional health. These are boundary issues where science and religion share common concerns. Both are joined at the boundaries between them. A fourth relationship is one of integration. Here mysticism and science are integrated (Sagar, 2002). The neurological study of the brain in terms of mystical and religious experiences indicates an integrative approach (d'Aquili and Newberg, 1998).

The third and fourth relationships dominate the study of spirituality in the health care research. A recent study indicates that there are over 2000 citations in three health care databases on spirituality's effect on health (O'Connor et al., 2002). Health care researchers other than chaplains carried out a vast majority of these studies. They include nursing, internal medicine, cardiology, neurology, pediatrics, family medicine, OT/PT, social work, recreational therapy, etc. These other health care disciplines seek to integrate spirituality into their theory and practice, using evidence from research. These health care disciplines are using scientific means to provide evidence for addressing patient spirituality in treatment. This research on spirituality does not believe that religion and science are opposed or belong in separate realms. They believe that there is enough commonality between religion and science that they can join and be integrated. There are exceptions to this view in the health care literature and critiques of this development (Sloan et al., 1999; Sloan et al., 2000). However, could chaplaincy appreciate and utilize this evidence-based approach to spirituality?

3. TRADITION-DRIVEN CHAPLAINCY UTILIZES EVIDENCE

There is an assumption that faith does not require evidence. However, within the Christian tradition, faith and evidence are not mutually exclusive. Murray Elkin in his Foreword to *Randomized Controlled Trials* (Jadad, 1999) notes that Daniel, the prophet, performed the earliest clinical trial (Dan. 1: 8-17). Daniel set up a ten-day trial comparing the health effects of a vegetarian diet on himself and his companions with the health effect of the royal Babylonian diet on the other boys. The vegetarian diet proved more beneficial. The guard overseeing the trial believed the evidence and gave Daniel and his companions only a vegetarian diet. Elkin notes that this clinical trail would not meet today's standards especially with divine intervention as a confounding variable! In a similar clinical trial, the prophet Elijah challenges the prophets of Baal to show evidence of their god (1Kings 18: 20-40). The success of Elijah's trial led the Israelite people to a deeper faith in God. Both these examples from the Hebrew Bible indicate that the prophets Daniel and Elijah were not afraid of the evidence. In fact, they used evidence to build faith.

In the Christian Bible, the healing stories of Jesus are evidence of his power and identity and can lead to faith (Pilch, 1997). Thomas the Apostle requires strong evidence before he will believe in the post-Resurrection Jesus. He says: "Unless I see the holes that the nails made in his hands and can put my finger into the holes they made, and unless I can put my hand into his side, I refuse to believe" (Jn. 20: 25). Thomas wants concrete evidence to believe that Jesus has risen. The evidence that he sees and critically reviews leads to deeper faith.

Most faith groups today require some evidence to indicate that a person has been called to ministry. The call to ministry is not just an internal, mystical awareness. The call to ministry is also evidenced in the life of the person and the work that he/she does. The evidence comes in various forms: psychological tests, seminary reports, academic grades, field placement reports, CPE units, letters of reference, examination by a ministry committee, etc. There are various forms of evidence that faith groups utilize to evaluate the call to ministry of a candidate.

In health care chaplaincy, the clinical method is a crucial form of evidence that guides the chaplain. While chaplaincy historically has based its mandate on the tradition of the faith group, evidence is part of the ministry. From a Christian perspective, for example, many chaplains offer pastoral care for the sick because the Scriptures tell them to do so. Christian chaplains and pastors believe that Christ wants them to care for the sick "for what so ever you do to the least, you do unto Christ" (Mt. 25:40). Caring for the sick has been a rich and long part of the tradition. However, the tradition of pastoral care is not devoid of evidence. Chaplains offer care because of the tradition and because it is helpful to the person in need (Wise, 1966). If the clinical experience indicates that the person who is sick is not benefiting from the pastoral care, then usually the chaplain/pastor will change the care or stop it. Such a decision is based on clinical evidence. According to evidence-based health care, this is level 2 evidence. Thus, while chaplaincy is historically more tradition driven, there are some levels of evidence that are part of the practice of ministry. VandeCreek (1995) has researched and assembled much evidence for the importance of chaplains and spirituality in the care of patients. However, how much of this evidence-based approach is utilized by chaplains?

4. SPIRITUALITY IS THE DOMAIN OF CHAPLAINCY AND WE OUGHT TO USE THE EVIDENCE OR LOSE OUR LEADERSHIP

The role of chaplaincy is the cure of souls (MacNeill, 1951; Clebsch and Jaeckle, 1967; Holifield, 1983; O'Connor, 1999b; Oden, 1984). Chaplaincy has a rich tradition based on caring for the sick and facilitating the cure of souls. Dante in the *Divine Comedy* (Paradise, 1962, XVII, 20) believed that the cure of souls took place as the soul was purged of sin through grace in climbing Mount Purgatory (Dante, Purgatory, 1955; O'Connor, 1999b). The focus of chaplaincy in caring for the spiritual, soul needs of the sick has proved its worth. The other health care disciplines are now seeing this as essential. These other disciplines have taken it one step further and have been engaged in doing scientific research on spirituality and health (Koenig, 1997). This research has produced two trends. One is that spirituality can be an effective coping method for challenging health care situations (Levin et al.,

1997). This means that one's faith, spiritual practices, beliefs, etc., can help the person and family deal with situations that are difficult or impossible to change (Pargament, 1997). Examples are geriatrics (Koenig and Weaver, 1998), palliative care (O'Connor, 1998) and disability (O'Connor, 1999a; Meakes et al., 2002). The other trend is that spirituality can at times be a determinant of health. This means that spiritual practices, beliefs, faith, etc., can positively influence health (Bryd, 1988; Levin et al., 1997; O'Laoire, 1997; Harris et al., 1999). This has more mixed results (Astin et al., 2000) and has received more criticism (Sloan et al., 1999; Sloan et al., 2000).

Interestingly, non-chaplains conduct this research. These non-chaplains are developing a theory and research base for spirituality and taking the leadership in the field (VandeCreek, 1999; O'Connor, 2000; O'Connor et al., 2002). Investigators in other disciplines have taken over research on spirituality and chaplains are the followers. It is easy to imagine in the near future when a nurse who specializes in spirituality will be teaching courses to chaplains on spirituality in health care using the research in the field.

The strengths of health care chaplaincy are its clinical training and experience in the field. Chaplains through Clinical Pastoral Education (CPE) have learned to address the spiritual needs in patients in an ecumenical and interfaith context. CPE educates chaplains not to impose their spirituality on patients but hear the patients' spiritual narratives and seek to respond within those narratives. I have been asked by many nurses, doctors and other therapists how to address and respond to patients' spiritual concerns. My quick answer is: "Take a CPE unit and you will begin to learn!" At the same time, I have said to these same health care professionals and researchers: "Teach us how to read, understand, critique and implement the research evidence on spirituality into our clinical practice. Teach us how to do research on spirituality." Chaplaincy needs to be more evidence based to be leaders in our area of expertise (O'Connor and Meakes, 1998; O'Connor, 2000).

CONCLUSION

Chaplaincy ought to be more scientific and evidence based in its ministry. The evidence is already there in the health care databases and ought to be utilized. This is the search for truth that is at the very basis of theology and chaplaincy. In the post-modern world, theology and medical science have realized that truth is more complex than previously understood. Truth is pluralistic and ambiguous (Tracy, 1987). A variety of scientific methods such as quantitative, qualitative, case study, and clinical wisdom are needed. Similarly a variety of theological methods using sacred texts, traditions, poetry, literature, mystical experiences, and faith are also needed in the search for truth. All of these constitute various forms of evidence.

At the same time, I do not believe that if chaplaincy becomes more scientific that it will preserve and/or augment our place in health care reform. The key to the position of chaplaincy is not necessarily solid evidence that shows our worth but that those in administration value the role of chaplaincy. Here at Hamilton Health Sciences, the chaplaincy department is being scaled back because of budget cuts. We have provided empirical evidence to show our worth. However, the administration maintains its position even with the evidence. In the same geographical area, a religious hospital is increasing the number and role of chaplaincy. The reason for this increase is that chaplaincy is part of their mission statement, part of their values. While I advocate chaplaincy becoming more scientific in its pursuit of truth, I also realize that it will not necessarily save our jobs. However, looking back on my encounter with the physician in 1992, I would now answer: "We walk in the paradox of both faith and evidence."

REFERENCES

Astin, J. A., Harkness, E., and Ernest, E. (2000). The efficacy of 'Distant Healing': A systematic review of randomized trials. *Annals of Internal Medicine* 132: 903-910.

Barbour, I. (1997). *Religion and science: Historical and contemporary issues.* San Francisco: Harper-Collins.

Bryd, R. (1988). Positive therapeutic effects of intercessory prayer in a coronary care unit population. *Southern Medical Journal* 81(7), 826-829.

Clebsch, W. & Jaeckle, C. R. (1967). *Pastoral care in historical perspective.* New York: Harper.

Dante, A. (1955). *The Divine Comedy* Purgatory, D. Sayers (trans.) London: Penguin.

Dante, A. (1962). *The Divine Comedy* Paradise, D. Sayers and B. Reynolds (trans.) London: Penguin.

D'Aquili, E. & Newberg, A. B. (1999). *The mystical mind: Probing the biology of religious experience.* Minneapolis: Fortress Press.

Donald, A. (1992). *Evidence-based medicine: A report from McMaster medical school and teaching hospitals.* Anglia and Oxford health Authorities; Brisbane, Australia.

Gartner, J., Larson, D., and Vachar-Mayberry, C. (1990). A Systematic Review of the Quantity and Quality of Empirical Research Published in Four Pastoral Counseling Journals. *The Journal of Pastoral Care* 44, (2), Summer, 115-123.

Harris, W. S., Gowda, M., Kolb, J., Strychacz, C., Vacek, J. L, Jones, P. G., Forker, A., O'Keefe, J. H., and McCallister, B. D. (1999). A randomized controlled trial of the effects of remote, intercessory prayer on outcomes in patients admitted to a coronary unit. *Archives of Internal Medicine* vol. 159, Oct. 25 1999, 2273-2278.

Holifield, E. B. (1983). *A history of pastoral care in America.* Nashville: Abingdon Press.

Ignatieff, M. (2000). *The Rights Revolution.* Toronto: Ansani Press.

Jadad, A. (1999). *Randomized control trials.* London: British Medical Journal.

Koenig, H. (1997). *Is religion good for your health: The effects of religion on physical and mental health.* New York: The Haworth Press, Inc.

Koenig, H. and Weaver, A. (1998). *Pastoral care of older adults.* Minneapolis, MN: Fortress Press.

Lancet, September 23 1995, Editorial p. 785.

Levin, J. S., Larson, D. B., and Puchalski, C. M., (1997). Religion and spirituality in medicine: Research and education. *JAMA* Spetember 3, 278(9), 792-793.

MacNeill, T. (1951). *A history of the cure of souls.* New York: Harper.

Marks, S. (1999). Qualitaitve Studies. *PDQ Evidence-based principles and practice.* A. McKibbon (ed.) Hamilton: BC Decker, 187-204.

Mays, N., and Pope, C. (1995). Rigour and qualitative research. *British Medical Journal* 311 July 8, 109-112.

McKibbon, A. (1999). *PDQ Evidence-based principles and practice.* Hamilton: B.C. Decker.

Meakes, E., O'Connor, T., and Carr, S. (2002). The great leveler: Gender and the Institutionalized Disabled on Faith and Disability, *Journal of Religion, Disability and Health* (in press).

O'Connor T., Meakes, E., McCaroll-Butler, P., Gadowsky, S. and O'Neill, K. (1997). Making the most and making sense: Ethnographic research on spirituality in palliative care *The Journal of Pastoral Care* Spring, 51(1), 25-36.

O'Connor, T. & Meakes, E. (1998). Hope in the midst of challenge: Evidence-based pastoral care. *The Journal of Pastoral Care* 52(4) Winter, 359-368.

O'Connor, T., O'Neill, K., Rao, V., van der Zyl, M., McKinnon, S., Roadhouse, J., Meakes, E. and van de Laar, T. (1999a). Horse of a different color: Ethnography of faith and disability. *The Journal of Pastoral Care* 53, (3), Fall, 269-284.

O'Connor, T. (1999b). Climbing Mt Purgatory: Dante's cure of souls and contemporary narrative therapy. *Pastoral Psychology* 47, 6, 445-457.

O'Connor, T. (2000). Response to Larry VandeCreek: Brief communication. *The Journal of Pastoral Care* 54, (2), 2000, 217-218.

O'Connor, T., McCarroll-Butler, P., Meakes, E., Jadad, A. and Davis, A. (2002). Review of quantity and types of spirituality research in three health care databases (1962-1999): What are the implications for health care ministry? *The Journal of Pastoral Care* Summer 56(2) (in press).

O'Laoire, S. (1997). An experimental study of the effects of distant, intercessory prayer on self-esteem, anxiety and depression. *Alternative Therapeutic Health Medicine* 1997, 3, 38-53.

Paragment, K. (1997). *Psychology of religion and coping*. New York: Guilford Press.

Oden, T. (1984). *The care of souls in the classic tradition*. Philadelphia: Fortress Press.

Pilch, J. (1997). *Healing in the new testament*. Minneapolis, MN: Fortress Press.

Rosenberg, W. and Donald, A. (1992). Evidence-based medicine: An approach to clinical problem-solving. *British Medical Journal* 310, April, 1122-5.

Sagar, S. (2002). *Restored harmony: An evidence based approach for integrating traditional Chinese medicine into complementary cancer care*. Hamilton, ON: Dreaming Dragonfly Communications.

Sloan, R., Bagiela, E. and Powell, T. (1999). Religion, spirituality and medicine. *The Lancet*, 353, February 20, 664-667;

Sloan, R., Bagiella, E., VandeCreek, L., Hover, M., Casalone, C., Hirsch, T., Hasan, Y., Kreger, R. and Poulos, P. (2000). Sounding board: Should physicians prescribe religious activities. *The New England Journal of Medicine*, 342(25), June 22, 1913-1916.

Tracy, D. (1987). *Plurality and ambiguity* New York: Harper and Row.

VandeCreek, L. (ed.) (1995). *Spiritual needs and pastoral services: Readings in research*. Decatur, Georgia: Journal of Pastoral Care Publications.

VandeCreek, L. (1999). Professional chaplaincy: An absent profession. *The Journal of Pastoral Care* 53 (4), Winter, 417-432.

Wise, C. (1966). *The meaning of pastoral care*. New York: Harper and Row.

Health Care Reform: Opportunities for Professional Chaplains to Build Intentional Communities of Learners by Integrating Faith, Science, Quality, and Systems Thinking

Bartholomew Rodrigues, MDiv, MA, BCC

SUMMARY. Albert Einstein once said, "The significant problems we face cannot be solved at the same level of thinking we were at when we created them" (www.brainyquote.com). Health care reform has brought professional chaplains to a place of chaos–a place that raises many questions about the past, present and future. This chaos presents tremendous opportunities for professional chaplains to increase their capacities in building intentional communities of learners by integrating faith, science, quality and systems thinking. Pastoral care givers must truly understand the pressures from all sides and the new emerging paradigm of integrated health care delivery. Without this understanding, we will not see the opportunities and challenges of integrating pastoral and spiritual care in the emerging structures and systems. The future of chaplaincy

---

Bartholomew Rodrigues is Director of Mission, Ethics/Integrity and Spiritual Care, Providence Health System, Medford, OR 97504-6225 (E-mail: brodrigues@providence.org).

[Haworth co-indexing entry note]: "Health Care Reform: Opportunities for Professional Chaplains to Build Intentional Communities of Learners by Integrating Faith, Science, Quality, and Systems Thinking." Rodrigues, Bartholomew. Co-published simultaneously in *Journal of Health Care Chaplaincy* (The Haworth Pastoral Press, an imprint of The Haworth Press, Inc.) Vol. 13, No. 1, 2002, pp. 195-211; and: *Professional Chaplaincy and Clinical Pastoral Education Should Become More Scientific: Yes and No* (ed: Larry VandeCreek) The Haworth Pastoral Press, an imprint of The Haworth Press, Inc., 2003, pp. 195-211. Single or multiple copies of this article are available for a fee from The Haworth Document Delivery Service [1-800-HAWORTH, 9:00 a.m. - 5:00 p.m. (EST). E-mail address: docdelivery@haworthpress.com].

10.1300/J080v13n01_04   *195*

largely will depend on the quality of the data, quality of our conversations and our ability to thinking together through dialogue. *[Article copies available for a fee from The Haworth Document Delivery Service: 1-800-HAWORTH. E-mail address: <docdelivery@haworthpress.com> Website: <http://www.HaworthPress.com> © 2002 by The Haworth Press, Inc. All rights reserved.]*

KEYWORDS. Chaplain, pastoral care, chaplaincy, health care reform, managed care

The limits of chaplaincy leadership are being tested by our ability to see clearly and lead wisely. The leadership is challenged not only to provide resources for hands on ministry but also resources for chaplains to develop systems thinking which will ensure the future of chaplaincy. The two professions–clinical pastoral education and professional chaplaincy need to become more scientific in response to health care reform. They have done a very good job in integrating faith to pastoral theology and practices, but they need to develop tools and practices to integrate science, quality, and systems thinking. They need to give attention and priority to testing our health care ministries by scientific studies, by examining the nature and scope of services provided, establish baselines, thresholds, benchmarks and develop ways to improve these ministries based on results. Scientific investigation and data can help chaplains to be better engaged in thinking together through the process of dialogue–dialogue with our administrators, sponsors, and community who can be advocates for an expanded vision of pastoral and spiritual care.

How can pastoral care professionals be on the cutting edge of tomorrow's ministry? The future of clinical chaplaincy largely will depend on the quality of the data, quality of our conversations and our ability of thinking together through dialogue. Besides, there is a growing interest and a need to demonstrate how professional chaplaincy encounters help the patient's healing and recovery process, and why professional clinical chaplaincy services need to be established, maintained, and integrated. Albert Einstein once said, "The significant problems we face cannot be solved at the same level of thinking we were at when we created them" (www.brainyquote.com) Health care reform has brought us, as clinical professional chaplains to a place of chaos–a place, which raises a whole lot of questions about the past, present and future. This chaos presents tremendous opportunities for professional clinical chaplains to increase our capacities in building intentional communities of learners by integrating faith, science, quality and systems thinking. Clinical pastoral care givers must truly understand the pressures from all sides and the new emerging paradigm of integrated health care delivery. Without this understanding, we will not see the opportunities and challenges of integrating pastoral and spiritual care in the emerging structures and systems.

HEALTH CARE REFORM–INVISIBLE, BUT NOT SILENT

Who has seen the wind?
Neither I nor you:
But when the leaves hang trembling
The wind is passing through

Who has seen the wind?
Neither you nor I:
But when the trees bow down their heads
The wind is passing by.

The poet Christina Rossetti reminds us (Rossetti, 1893) how susceptible we are to the influence of unseen forces. At one moment, the gentle wind may help us relax and unwind; at another moment, the wind can be violent, angry and brutal. Invisible but not silent, the wind has the capacity to rustle leaves, lift kites, carry seeds, power sails, and support wings. It can destroy homes, uproot trees, and down power lines. The wind can be unpredictable and terrifying; it can also be life giving, and renewing.

Continuing the metaphor, anyone who has experienced health care reform in the last decade knows what it is to be buffeted and shaped by powerful but sometimes unseen forces from every side. We could liken the pressures to winds from the four compass points (see Figure 1).

From the Far East, health care faced the pressures of more accountability a need for quality control and improvement (some examples: reducing errors, reducing medical waste and inefficiency). From the West there are pressures for private good at the cost of common good, technology explosion, and the use of the latest new medical technology. From the north and top come powerful economic interests of restraining cost by providing incentives to individuals and providers for effective and economical use of limiting

FIGURE 1. Health Care Reform: The Four Compass Points

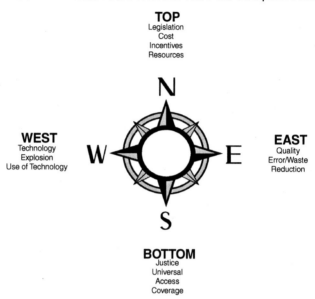

TOP
Legislation
Cost
Incentives
Resources

WEST
Technology
Explosion
Use of Technology

EAST
Quality
Error/Waste
Reduction

BOTTOM
Justice
Universal
Access
Coverage

resources, and non-beneficial treatment. From the south and bottom are voices for justice, universal access, equity, and adequate health care.

I. THE "FAR-EAST WINDS" ARE THE FORCES OF QUALITY CONTROL AND PROCESS IMPROVEMENT

In order for clinical professional chaplains to secure a firm place it would seem that a quality focus and a strong research base is imperative because quality care is not driven solely by the professional integrity of health care providers; rather quality is demanded and defined by health care consumers and is central to patient-centered care. To survive within the competitive health care market, quality is a priority initiative for most health care organizations. Clinical chaplaincy services perform variety of roles in today's complex health care systems. Through its quality initiative programs within its institution, chaplains can demonstrate how value-added the services rendered are. These roles and the expectations associated with them must be clear to everyone involved. Unclear or confusing roles result in decreased use of pastoral services, fewer referrals, less participation on committees, and diminished credibility within the institution.

Administrators and decision-makers need to know to what extent chaplains meet the needs and expectations of the many customers who make up the health care context. It is important that departments and institutions define important aspects of spiritual care–its indicators of quality, collect, and evaluate those key factors and data elements. It also must include specific questions on chaplaincy services through patient satisfaction instruments. There are some very good models available (VandeCreek, 1997). Doing so would demonstrate its role alongside other professionals in emphasizing quality care. It would also demonstrate how spiritual care fits into the hospital care plan as a whole. Besides, the Joint Commission on Accreditation of Healthcare Organizations (Joint Commission) requires interdisciplinary performance improvement activities to ensure continuous quality improvement.

How long will institutions that seriously attempt to address the holistic character of a patient's well being be able to commit to making a commitment to providing clinical chaplaincy services? How long will it be an essential element of their mission and identity? Chaplains rely on their CEOs or the person who their department reports to for spiritual care advocacy and services. Is it true, as has been suggested (CHA, 1990) that clinical chaplaincy position on administrative charts is frequently more by reputation than proven value? But, why should pastoral care endeavors be initiated and shaped by others' perceptions? Clinical professional chaplaincy services budgets need to be proven by value rather than by mere sponsorship and reputation of mission and identity of an institution. Is it necessary to demonstrate optimal delivery of this care through scientific investigation and quality improvement initiatives? Having empirical data can only strengthen the need for clinical professional chaplaincy services during times of high economic pressure. Clinical professional chaplaincy services should not be exempt from the scrutiny of science nor should it rest on its laurels but keep pace with the demands of the new evolving health care paradigm. Science and Faith should work together.

As clinical professional chaplaincy finds itself evolving as an integrated discipline into the total interdisciplinary health care continuum, it needs the scrutiny like any other department and discipline in healthcare to show that its services provide a measurable, significant outcome. If the services provided are measurable and provide significant outcomes, one direction might be in developing spiritual care services as a reimbursable service, like any other service. Chaplains need to help our religious sponsors and our health care institutions recover and sustain patient centered spiritual care–sustain a holistic treatment plan; treatment of body, mind and spirit. But, how does chaplaincy participate in the performance improvement initiative of the organization?

The FOCUS-PDCA or variations of it like FOCUS-PDSA methodologies, very common in hospitals, should help chaplaincy teams look at work as a series of processes. The letters in the model's name refer to the following nine steps:

- *F*ind a process that needs improvement, (Step 1)
- *O*rganize a team that knows the process, (Step 2)
- *C*larify current knowledge of the process, (Step 3)
- *U*nderstand the process and learn the causes of process variation, (Step 4)
- *S*elect the improvement opportunities, (Step 5)
- *P*lan the test of the selected improvement, (Step 6)
- *D*o the test and collect data for analysis, (Step 7)
- *C*heck the results, or Study the Results–did the test validate or contradict the theory? (Step 8 and Step 9)
- *A*ct upon the results–either implement the improvement or go back to Step 5.

Chaplains can also use part of the above tool (like PDCA cycle only) for their day-to-day use or join other teams who use a similar process. SWOT analysis can also help chaplains work through all the information needed. "SWOT" stands for strengths, weaknesses, opportunities, and threats. Using SWOT components as a basis for action strategies can be developed and implemented. Methodologies such as these are meant to improve a process in incremental stages.

The Chaplaincy profession needs to increasingly seek and demonstrate that its practice is based on sound scientific principles validated by rigorous research, in other words that its practice is evidence-based. Evidence-based practice requires not only carefully evaluated interventions judged through objective criteria (such as quality improvement methodologies like FOCUS-PDCA, FOCUS-PDSA), but also input from patients in a systematic way that provides a foundation for patient-centered care. Consideration of both (input from patients and evidence) are essential if the best outcomes of chaplaincy intervention are to ensue. Evidence-based approaches utilize systematic thinking approach and chaplains need to be familiar with the science of Systems Thinking (Senge, 1990), Dialogue (Isaacs, 1999) and inquiry. It is imperative that chaplains produce verifiable evidence of its services while mounting a critique of the evidence-based movement as well. Science and Faith should work together. Spiritual and pastoral care needs and services must be viewed scientifically even though chaplains may have few compelling reasons to let research results influence their work (VandeCreek, 1995). Clinical professional chaplaincy is not only an art but a science as well–it is a matter of heart, spirit, and mind. The voice of caring, the voices of science and research (qualitative and quantitative) need to have voices at the table of dialogue and process improvement. Science can establish credibility through research, in so far, as quality improvement and outcomes become part and parcel of chaplaincy services. Science and faith should work together particularly when it is necessary to demonstrate optimal delivery of care.

II. OUR "WEST WINDS" ARE THE TECHNOLOGICAL ADVANCEMENTS IN SOCIETY AND MEDICINE

These winds bring tremendous improvements and convenience but also a degree of depersonalization. Advanced technology has enhanced our ability to diagnose and treat critically ill patients, thereby assisting in prolonging life for many. However, its high cost has been prohibitive, imposing more burdens than benefits on many patients (example: end-of-life care). Although technological advances have accelerated social change, many have also fuelled legal and ethical concerns. There are pressures to do everything possible to keep a person alive–happening both at the beginning of life, and at the end of life.

Medical science explodes with ingenuity, yet the public's ability to fund this inventiveness is severely limited. Competition using advance medical technological at high prohibitive cost imposes more burdens than benefits not only on patients as consumers but also burdens on health care providers and on scare community resources. Our nation's economy can no longer fully afford all the health care that medical science can bring us. The personal and pastoral aspects of medical practice, which are probably more important in helping patients toward health than we realize, are becoming increasingly stifled by health care systems, which are increasingly scientific, technological, and efficient. Clinical practice requires pastoral as well as technical skills, art as well as science, and yet the balance of current medical culture increasingly favors and encourages science over art.

Dying patients and their families repeatedly express their need for supports based on compassion and caring, yet healthcare efforts focus on often-ineffective technological interventions and procedures (O'Connell, 1996). The laudable successes of technological medical care unfortunately have further masked the inevitability of death in a culture that fails to accept death as an integral part of life (Super & Plutko, 1996). The "let's do everything possible" attitude that prevailed during the past few decades is both inhumane and wasteful. In contrast, in the new era of managed care with its focus on bottom line margin, a well-meaning physician may become suspect whenever he or she recommends against a medical intervention that is deemed futile (Basta & Tauth, 1996).

> Without health of the spirit, high technology focused strictly on the body offers limited hope for healing the whole person . . . A person may forgo extraordinary or disproportionate means of preserving life. Disproportionate means are those that in the patient's judgment do not offer a reasonable hope of benefit or entail an excessive burden, or impose excessive expense on the family or the community. (USCCB, 2001)

High-technology care must be balanced with a humanistic approach to meet the needs of the "whole person." Humanistic care needs to be fostered by cultivating open dialogue among patients, families, physicians, nurses, and other involved staff. Professional Chaplains can be agents and facilitators of this change by being involved in strategic planning, and internal or external community needs assessment committees. They can also be part of technology assessment committees, interdisciplinary care teams, and organizational ethics committee balance competing needs (example: preferential option for the poor on one end and high expensive piece of technology that caters to only a few). Chaplains need to have a role in reviewing resources allocations.

III. THE WINDS FROM UP NORTH ARE THE FORCES OF LEGISLATION; COST CUTTING MEASURES; DECLINING REIMBURSEMENT; AND HIGH ECONOMIC PRESSURES

Budget cuts and resulting changes in health care and its structuring have forced hospitals to change the way they deliver care. Our nation's healthcare system serves too few and costs too much. The winds of health care reform represent an effort to redirect a seventh of our national economy to reshape society's response to basic human need. It has touched every family, business, and every community.

There is a disturbing trend for health care systems to provide declining financial resources for spiritual care departments even while the spirituality movement is growing rapidly in the United States because of reduced operating margins and other factors. The decline in funding prompted Providence Health System to undertake ongoing research in Spiritual Care and Chaplaincy Services, to explore the nature and the role of chaplaincy services in healthcare settings (Rodrigues et al., 2000). Recent research studies are demonstrating a clearer link between spirituality and health. However, it remains a challenge for many healthcare organizations including those that are mission and faith-based hospitals to weave and integrate spirituality into organizational life and to make it an integral component of medical care. Organizations grounded in mission and spirituality have a tremendous opportunity to ensure that spirituality and mission will be the core of healthcare services, instead of parallel to or ornamental part ('looks-good-to-have' services) of clinical approaches. Linking spirituality with medicine and ensuring it becomes an integral part of interdisciplinary team agenda as well can be difficult because medical professionals and spiritual caregivers speak different languages. The focuses and expertises are different. To overcome these barriers clinical pastoral care professionals need to participate more actively in interdisciplinary team meetings also known as case conferences to exchange information on physical, emotional, and spiritual care of patients.

Religion and medicine were once closely linked, but spiritual concerns have come to be seen as obstacles to scientific progress or, at best, sentimental attachments of little real value in the battle with disease (Astrow et al., 2001). The public has shown increasing interest in the interplay of religion, spirituality, and health, but many physicians are either openly skeptical or unsure how best to respond. In the year 2002 Providence Health System was scheduled to follow up with a research study on physician perception and utilization of clinical chaplaincy services. Guiding patients to health takes more than technological wizardry, wonder drugs, and pleasantly decorated surroundings. In fact, to an increasing number of institutions, faith is the missing ingredient–faith in God or higher power, faith in oneself, faith in the possibilities for recovery (Hudson, 1996). Managed care and health care reform may be more on the anthropology and the ethics of pastoral care than the machinery for delivering health care (Maes, 1996).

In an environment of cost cutting measures, declining reimbursement and high economic pressures justification for clinical professional chaplaincy services requires accountability–accountability for its services and its effectiveness. Departments that do not continually clarify what they do, and how they do it, and establish baselines and thresholds of performance, may dangerously limit their continuity; let alone effectiveness. Chaplains can no longer hide behind their ministerial identity and ordination. Today's patients and administrators ask not only for compassion but also for competency. Chaplains need to develop new sets of skill and competencies that supersedes ordination and religious formation, and even one could say certification process for chaplains as well. Clinical pastoral education need to address the changing health care paradigm and incorporate new topics, such as research in pastoral care, methodologies in quality initiatives like FOCUS-PDCA, FOCUS-PDSA, focused dialogue on difficult issues utilizing *Dialogue and the Art of Thinking Together* (William Isaacs, 1999); *The Fifth Discipline* (Peter Senge,1990); and *Systems Thinking* (Daniel Kim, 1999).

IV. THE WINDS FROM BELOW (SOUTH) ARE THE VOICES OF JUSTICE FOR UNIVERSAL ACCESS, EQUITY, AND ADEQUATE HEALTH CARE COVERAGE

Though there are triumphal strides in medical advances, the American society has yet to ensure that each person has access to affordable health care. To correct this injustice, professional clinical chaplains can take a central role in health care reform and call on the nation's political and corporate leaders, including their department heads and pastoral care administrators, providers, and faith-based groups to join all Americans in a new national conversation on systemic health care reform. The ministry is one that compels both a proclamation to ministry values and a commitment to speak out against the challenges or threats to what are essential to the well-being of individuals and society.

Often times, physicians and family members hang too long on technological interventions–when the burden of a treatment has outweighed its potential benefits. The fear of litigation has also reinforced a tendency on the part of healthcare providers to persevere with aggressive medical therapy even when it is clearly futile. In such situations, chaplains can take a central role and provide spiritual direction, guidance, and ethical deliberations. Yet data from a national study (Rodrigues et al., 2000) suggests that chaplains continue to have a 'non-agenda'

(VandeCreek, 1997) stance. Chaplaincy ministry must be both a voice for the voiceless and an agent of transformation when there are competing and incompatible interests.

> Physicians want to retain or restore autonomy of practice. Hospitals want market choices but protection from market discipline. Suppliers of medical devices and pharmaceuticals want the widest range of proprietary control in the development and marketing of products and drugs. Insurers want release from cost shifting and mandated benefits and freedom to exclude high-risk individuals. Patients and consumers of health insurance want the greatest range of coverage at the lowest cost and access to the highest quality of medical care–without gatekeepers, waiting lists, or rationing of care. American taxpayers do not want to sacrifice the freedom represented by their disposable incomes, and many are reluctant to abandon unhealthy habits. In short . . . American health care is dominated by an individualism that asserts self- or group interest over the common good. (Dougherty, 1992)

Navigating the Wind Through Systems Thinking: Let us take a lesson from the successful sailor when we are tempted to believe our choices are limited, when we feel helpless and stranded with the many pressures and changes? The sailor makes a friend of the wind; buffeted by contrary breezes, the sailor chooses a tack and sets the sails; with one eye on the compass, the sailor strains forward towards the distant shore. To chart a solid course to the future, the two professions–clinical pastoral education and health care chaplaincy–should also endeavor to become more scientific by utilizing systems thinking. Systems thinking is a discipline of a learning organization which focuses on recognizing the interconnections between parts of a system, and how the parts are interrelated and interdependent on each other. Understanding how systems work and how chaplains play a role in them lets systems thinkers function more effectively and proactively. The more we understand systemic behavior the more we will be able to anticipate changes within and work with systems rather than be controlled by them. Chaplains need to build intentional community of system thinkers and be better designers of systems rather than mere operators in a system.

The circle of influence framework (see Figure 2) can help chaplains go beyond responding only as operators within a system, responding merely to events in a reactive mode but begin looking for actions with higher leverage as well. Events and day-to-day occurrences no doubt are

FIGURE 2. Circle of Influence Framework

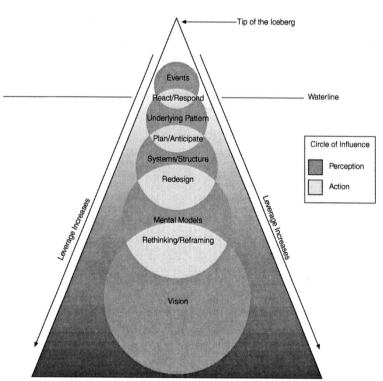

Adapted from Daniel H. Kim, Level of Perception

easily noticeable but are the results of deeper patterns and systemic structures, which are difficult to see like in an iceberg. The actions taken at higher levels will have more impact on future outcomes, not present events. Participating in quality improvement activities will help address the problems of health care reform from a higher leverage systemic perspective. It is time that chaplains create new systemic structures and take actions at the level of mental models by reflecting, contemplating by developing an ability to surface, suspend and question our own assumptions about how (health care) systems works and what is most important in the era of managed care.

Systems thinkers work from a central premise–if you don't know how you are producing certain outcomes, you'll have great difficulty determining how to produce better outcomes. Chaplains need to think together and sharpen their personal and collective insight to provocative questions such as, What structural causes might explain where we are today? Is the situation slowly getting worse? What new strategies need to be adopted and implemented? How long will the strategy or solution last? What new problem will the solution create? Using systems thinking, pastoral care professionals will have to think in new ways and envision a new future for the role of chaplaincy within the ministry.

Pressures can be very compelling because they often require an instant response. For example, if a house is burning, we react immediately by putting out the fire. Putting out the fire is an appropriate action, but if we do not analyze from a systemic perspective or take a deeper look, as to what might have caused the fire, chances are there will be another fire someday. Systems thinking not only views events and adaptive patterns but also analyzes underlying systemic structures, assumptions, and vision (Kim, 1999). Chaplains too by virtue of their roles have devoted time and resources on reactive (events) often at the neglect of inquiry, tempted too easily only on hands on ministry. Chaplains need to carve out time and balance action with contemplation, balance action with inquiry, balance faith with reason, and balance hands on ministry with reflection and learning. Jesus not only brought healing to persons in need, but he also healed those social structures of his day that impeded compassionate responses to the needs of persons. This, too, is a challenge and opportunity for organizations as well as chaplains. Caught between the security of the past and the ambiguity of the future chaplains find themselves in three camps.

> The first group is nostalgic for the 'golden age of chaplaincy.' These chaplains see themselves as the last of a revered generation of pastoral professionals. Fearing the uncertainty of the future, they spend their energies in retrenchment. In the second group are chaplains who, although more helpful, nevertheless admit they face an uphill battle. In the midst of discouragement, they realize that others are shaping their future. And then there is the third group. These chaplains feel that the changing ministry presents them with an unparalleled opportunity, restricted only by their own lack of imagination. They see this opportunity as both a burden and a blessing. These spiritual caregivers embrace the chaos and actively seek out new ways to offer others the healing power of Jesus. (CHA, 1997-b)

The CHA-NACC 1996 survey (CHA, 1997-a) shows that the pastoral care staff is entrenched in the illness model of acute care settings and not enough attention is given to the spiritual dimension of wellness and their role in the community. Results in another 1999 study (VandeCreek, 2000) suggest that pastoral care staff adopting strategies like placing pressure on administration, getting more involved in interdisciplinary and taking responsibility for additional activities. In order to apply pressure of any kind on any decision makers one would assume data, in terms of utilizations and outcomes in chaplaincy, would be critical.

Systems' thinking can help clinical professional chaplains to be seen as community resources and not only as hospital resources. It will enable chaplains to define their role both inside and outside the hospital walls and enable partnership with parish/congregational nurses, area clergy, health and human services agencies, crises/disaster response teams, community based support groups, drug and alcohol treatment programs, physician office, clinics, and Samaritan counseling centers. It is imperative that chaplains and their administrators see the role of clinical chaplains as community resources and not only as hospital resources. Their roles should be defined not only in a reactive-illness model in acute care settings but also in a proactive model in community settings as well. Ideally, faith communities should be centers for care, healing, and wellness, with hospitals as extensions of those communities.

CONCLUSION

The need to integrate faith and science, the need to utilize quality and systems thinking–seeing patterns in what we do, how we do, who it impacts and so on is greater than ever before. In organizations that use systems thinking–learning organizations–leaders see how the parts of a whole relate to each other. Rather than reacting to events with short-term solutions, they solve problems by analyzing the organization's or system's underlying patterns and structures. But in many organizations, crisis management is a way of life because there may not be resources dedicated for system thinking process, resources dedicated to slow down and to look at underlying patterns and trends or to review current practices and the underlying assumptions behind those practices. The quick fixes, which may yield some improvement, fail to get at the fundamental cause. Learning organizations' leaders must be willing to take the long view and not trade off long-term performance improvements for short-term gains.

Health care reform can be seen as a process of renewal. The process of renewal can free and empower us as we learn to eliminate irrelevant and outmoded practices noticed through quality improvement initiatives. The moment has come to ask–what kind of future can we as chaplains look forward to? The answer–our future–depends, as it always has, on how much we are willing to review critically the assumptions, models and structures under which we operate. Pastoral care departments will have to develop systems thinking capacity in order to navigate change.

Systems thinking can help chaplains and chaplaincy administrators to see patterns as they gain new insights and develop new strategies for results that would last. Systems thinking and research helps to create a more collective and visible mental model about important issues. Systems thinking can also help chaplains as well as chaplaincy administrators create an organizational and departmental cultural which encourages organizational and team learning, a culture that embraces change and complexity. Such thinking allows one to see how the parts of a whole relate to each other. Rather than reacting to events with short-term solutions, system thinking can solve problems by analyzing the organization's underlying patterns and structures.

Clinical professional chaplains need to play a central role in healthcare · reform by adjusting their sails and not just drifting along. Despite the winds buffeting in all directions, a direction still needs to be set. Our compass is our ministry most especially when we reflect the healing power of God's love and grace. We can only face forward in faith. Now it is time to look forward to the new paradigms, new leaders not only within our own circles and disciplines, but also beyond. We may not be able to direct the winds and may be even swimming against the tide of health care reform. Some chaos is inevitable when the wind blows where it will; so also the breath of the Spirit (Hebrew: *Rûah: spirit, wind, breath*). We need to understand that the Church's healing ministry necessitates letting go of the familiar in order to allow the yet uncreated newness to emerge. Let us invoke the Spirit-wind so that it may nudge us, strengthen us.

We perhaps may have to pray a different kind of prayer. A prayer to disturb us . . . most especially when our dreams have come true; when we have dreamed too little; when we arrived safely, because we sailed too close to shore. We may have to ask the Lord to disturb us, so that we may dare more boldly, to venture on wider seas, where only the storms will show the Lord's mastery. When losing sight of land, we may find faith in the stars. We may have to ask the Lord to push back the horizons of our hopes, and to push us in the future in strength, courage, and hope.

REFERENCES

Astrow AB., Puchalski CM., & Sulmasy DP. (2001). Religion, spirituality, and health care: Social, ethical, and practical considerations. *American Journal of Medicine, 110,* 283-287.

Basta, L. & Tauth, J. (1996). High technology near the end of life: Setting limits. *Journal of American College of Cardiology, 28,* 1623-1630.

CHA (1990). Quality Assurance & Pastoral Care: A Development and Implementation Guide, *Catholic Health Association,* p. ix.

CHA (1997-a). Chaplaincy: Moving Toward the Next Millennium. A Report of the Survey on the Status of Catholic Chaplaincy in Organized Systems of Healthcare, *Catholic Health Association.*

CHA (1997-b). Spiritual Care in a Community or Network Setting, *Catholic Health Association.*

Dougherty C. (1992). Ethical Values in Health Care Reform, *Journal of American Medical Association,* vol. 268, 1992, p. 2411.

Hudson T. (1996). Measuring the results of faith. *Hospital and Health Networks,* 70(18):22-28.

Isaacs, W. (1999). *A Pioneering Approach to Communicating in Business and in Life. Dialogue and the Art of Thinking Together.* (Doubleday, NY).

Kim DH. (1999). *Introduction to Systems Thinking,* (Pegasus, MA) p. 17.

Maes JL. (1996). Can pastoral counseling flourish in a world of managed care? *Journal of Pastoral Care*; 50(2):133-40.

O'Connell LJ. (1996). Changing the culture of dying. A new awakening of spirituality in America heightens sensitivity to needs of dying persons. *Health Progress,* 77, 16-20.

Rossetti C. (1893). *Sing-Song, A Nursery Rhyme Book,* (Macmillan, NY).

Rodrigues B. et al. (2000). *Spiritual Needs & Chaplaincy Services: A National Empirical Study on Chaplaincy Encounters in Health Care Settings,* (Providence Health System, Oregon).

Senge P. (1990). *The Fifth Discipline: The Art and Practice of the Learning Organization,* (Doubleday, New York City), pp. 9-12.

Super A. & Plutko LA. (1996). Danger signs. Coalition points to causes and consequences of inadequate care of the dying. *Health Progress,* 77, 50-54.

USCCB. (2001). Ethical and Religious Directives for Catholic Health Care Services, 2001 *United States Catholic Conference of Bishops,* (Washington, DC).

VandeCreek L., Bender H. & Jordon, MR. (1995). *Research in Pastoral Care and Counseling: Quantitative and Qualitative Approaches,* (Journal of Pastoral Care Publications, IL).

VandeCreek L. (1995). *Spiritual Needs and Pastoral Services; Readings in Research,* (Journal of Pastoral Care Publications, IL).

VandeCreek L. & Lyon, M. (1997). *Ministry of Hospital Chaplains: Patient Satisfaction,* (The Haworth Press, Inc., NY).
VandeCreek L. (2000). How Has Health Care Reform Affected Professional Chaplaincy Programs And How Are Department Directors Responding? *Journal of Healthcare Chaplaincy* 10(1):7-17.
www.brainyquote.com/quotes/quotes/a/q100658.html

The Chaplain as the Complete Philosopher

Orlo C. Strunk, Jr., PhD

SUMMARY. This paper argues that professional chaplaincy must reflect an authentic understanding of the religion and science dialogue by drawing not simply on the popular culture's views but on the long traditions of serious scholarship and research that explores both these worlds. The author claims that what often passes as science is really scientism or technophilia and that such distortions should not be allowed to guide or define the chaplain's or the clinical educator's healthcare ministry. The chaplain, as a reflection of religion, is obligated to draw on all of humankind's projects of enquiry–science, art, humanities, theological and religious studies, ethics–and ought not become a captive of a Zeitgeist that invites idolatry either in the forms of scientism and technophilia or in the forms of provincial and superficial understandings of religion. *[Article copies available for a fee from The Haworth Document Delivery Service: 1-800-HAWORTH. E-mail address: <docdelivery@haworthpress.com> Website: <http://www.HaworthPress.com> © 2002 by The Haworth Press, Inc. All rights reserved.]*

KEYWORDS. Chaplaincy, religion, science, research

Orlo C. Strunk, Jr. is a Pastoral Counselor and Editor of the *Journal of Pastoral Care & Counseling (E-mail:OrloS@aol.com).*

[Haworth co-indexing entry note]: "The Chaplain as the Complete Philosopher." Strunk, Orlo C., Jr. Co-published simultaneously in *Journal of Health Care Chaplaincy* (The Haworth Pastoral Press, an imprint of The Haworth Press, Inc.) Vol. 13, No. 1, 2002, pp. 213-221; and: *Professional Chaplaincy and Clinical Pastoral Education Should Become More Scientific: Yes and No* (ed: Larry VandeCreek) The Haworth Pastoral Press, an imprint of The Haworth Press, Inc., 2003, pp. 213-221. Single or multiple copies of this article are available for a fee from The Haworth Document Delivery Service [1-800-HAWORTH, 9:00 a.m. - 5:00 p.m. (EST). E-mail address: docdelivery@haworthpress.com].

10.1300/J080v13n01_05

Several years ago in response to an invitation to write a personal reflection on the topic of aging and spiritual growth, I titled the chapter "Positive Spins on Bad Ideas" (Weaver, Koenig, & Roe, 1998). I argued that growing old is basically a bad idea although one could, if pressed, detect a few positive spins to this developmental phase of life. One of the "spins" I noted was that as one enters the "twilight years," memory can sometimes provide a genuine perspectival aura that may help to understand and appreciate the complexity of many of life's issues, that it may also help one resist the tendency for premature closure regarding awfully complex issues, and that it can even offer a kind of soothing lotion in the form of the idea that "what goes around comes around."

These thoughts–and a few others I hope to note in this essay–floated into consciousness as I read the two perspectives regarding the possible role of a scientific stance in the future of clinical pastoral education and health care chaplaincy. For one thing, I found myself agreeing with both arguments–*yes*, chaplaincy of the future ought to be more scientific; *yes*, chaplaincy and clinical pastoral education ought not become overly concerned regarding the scientific paradigm, particularly as it is often heralded in the healthcare community, and should instead proclaim the voice of authentic religion.

Then memory and nostalgia broke in. I recalled my years as a graduate student when, serving as the part-time Executive Secretary of the Institute of Pastoral Care, I spent many hours listening and recording the Minutes of the Institute's Board as its members dialogued, sometimes downright argued, over attempts to identify the place of CPE in theological studies and in the formation of ministers. As a relatively young man–I was in my very early thirties at the time–I felt privileged to sit with such pioneers as Joe Fletcher, Paul Johnson, John Billinsky, Rollin Fairbanks, Jim Burns, Walter Muelder, to note but a sample.

For hours on end, these clinicians and academics would discuss such topics as: Should it be called clinical pastoral *training* or clinical pastoral *education?* Should the main emphasis of the movement be on developing *clinical* skills or on achieving *pastoral* presence? Would the best education and training in clinical centers be *psychoanalytic* or *client-centered* in orientation? Is the best learning context in the *general* hospital or the *mental* hospital? Who should administer this aspect of theological education–the *seminaries* or the *hospitals* or the *professional associations?* And so it went. And as anyone who has followed these and dozens of other matters in the history of clinical pastoral education and professional chaplaincy knows (e.g., Hall, 1992), the movement has managed to resolve such complex issues via a lively, if at times contentious, series of dialogues, conferences, committee meetings, etc.

What has become eminently clear to me in these twilight years is that most of those early dialogues and disagreements were about *assumptions*–those quiet meaning systems that feed and generate the positions we take on matters of policy and practice. I suspect the issue regarding the role of science in the future development of professional chaplaincy and clinical pastoral education is equally driven by assumptions–in this instance the assumptions we hold regarding science, religion, and chaplaincy.

SCIENCE

The late Harvard professor Gordon W. Allport began his classical treatment of the dilemma of science and the single case with the phrase "science is an arbitrary creed" (Allport, 1937, p. vii). It is as true a claim today as it was then, although contemporary understandings of science are made more complex by its being confused with technology and its homogenization with political and economic forces.

The notion of science as an arbitrary creed is made most palatable when one is reminded of our inevitable encapsulation as human beings. In this regard, I turn to another famous American scholar, William James, for guidance. In his classic *The Principles of Psychology*, James devotes an entire chapter on what he calls "sub-universes," those perspectives of reality characteristic of the human species. He identified seven such "worlds"–(1) the world of sense, (2) the world of science, (3) the world of ideal relations, (4) the world of "idols of the tribe," (5) the various supernatural worlds, (6) the various worlds of individual opinion, and (7) the worlds of "sheer madness and vagary" (James, 1950, chapter XXI).

Although there have been many other classification schema regarding perceptions of reality before and since James's elaboration, what seems especially significant for the topic of this essay is that such perspectives are *real* and that there is on the part of humans a marked tendency to claim one of the worlds as "ultimate reality." James also insisted that what he called the "complete philosopher" be able "to assign to every given object of his thought its right place in one or other of these sub-worlds, but he also seeks to determine the relation of each sub-world to the others in the total world which *is*" (p. 291)–a suggestion I will turn to later in discussing the identity of the contemporary professional chaplain.

What makes the current issue of the role of science especially problematic are at least three conditions: (1) the confusion of science with technology and the resulting technophilia, (2) the political and financial forces that often cloud and make superficial the purely science/religion dialogue, and (3) the propensity of the ruling paradigm to cannibalize other perspectives.

The first concern, scientism and technophilia, is rampant in popular culture but often spills into our professional work settings, including hospitals. After all, most contemporary professional chaplains surely must be enamored by the technological advancements surrounding them in the modern hospital. Yearning to be identified as part of this "scientific" community seems only a natural propensity. Yet, few chaplains and religiously-based pastoral caregivers have the education, training, or, I suspect, the temperament to fall comfortably within the "sub-universe" called science.

Secondly, science, including its expression in technology, does not exist in a vacuum. In institutions that wrap themselves in the scientific cloak–such as hospitals–political and financial forces are bound to develop. For despite the scientific platitude of "objectivity," no arbitrary creed escapes completely evangelistic zeal, however subtle it might be. Professional chaplains, on a day-to-day basis, are immersed in this world, even though, as I hope to imply throughout this essay, it is not their true home.

Finally, it is well to be alert to a well-known historic reality; namely, that the dominant worldview–whether it be science or religion–tends to cannibalize other world views. Sometimes this is an overt and even brutal process, particularly in the case of totalitarian regimes. More often than not, however, in our professional arena the propensity is a much more subtle enterprise, particularly if the dominant worldview finds itself pressured to include within its original creed those phenomena traditionally integral to other "worlds."

This possibility recently struck me as I read and re-read the "White Paper," that attempt to define the role and importance of professional chaplaincy in healthcare (VandeCreek & Burton, 2001). In that document, considerable effort is exerted in the endeavor to identify historic and contemporary healthcare chaplaincy with the expansion of a "scientific" project (medicine) with its newfound interest in spirituality–a factor not evident in that profession's strong connection to the world of science.

This growing interest in the attempt to embrace spirituality within the scientific paradigm creates conceptual issues of considerable immensity, although much of the dialogue has not been addressed at a level deserving of the rich conceptual modifications in science's foundational assumptions, especially in terms of its roots in logical positivism and empiricism. Medicine, including its expression in the broad field of mental health, often couches this expansion of its turf in terms of the recent "scientific" evidence that there appears to be enough empirical research to warrant such an admittance, although, as it has been amply demonstrated by serious researchers (e.g., Koenig, 1997), the empirical (read scientific) research does not actually demonstrate a particularly solid tie between spirituality and health. Rather, there is considerable empirical research linking religion and various healthcare issues (e.g., Larson, Swyers, & McCullough, 1998; Koenig, McCullough, & Larson, 2001).

But, again, the scientific world–particularly as it has evolved in the human sciences–has demonstrated decades of hostility toward religion and nearly a complete neglect of the research in religious experience and behavior. Even today as it attends to "spirituality," the scientific efforts systematically avoids referencing the long and rich history of research in the scientific study of religion, including and especially the massive research in the psychology of religion (Wulff, 1991).

This scotoma on the part of the scientific community remains evident by science's attempt to dilute religion by reconstructing its rich and authentic meanings. This massive reconstruction project is especially evident in the mental health movement which goes to great length to debase or at least limit religion to its institutional and provincial expressions, despite a voluminous literature in the area of religious and theological studies–a literature rarely acknowledged in the contemporary writing and research lauding the spirituality factor.

When chaplains and pastoral counselors–authentic representatives of the world of *religion*–join in this subterfuge they do considerable dis-service to both the intellectual integrity of religious and theological scholarship but also are in danger of overlooking patients' primary concerns and expressions for religious care.

In this regard, chaplains, by reasons of their theological and ethical education and their identity as religious professions, might better include in their intellectual concerns the critiquing of what passes for science rather than uncritically embracing its epistemological sovereignty. As Simone Weil put it many years ago, and as only she could put it, "The disappearance of scientific truth appears to our eyes as the disappearance of truth, thanks to our habit of mistaking the one for the other. So soon as truth disappears, utility at once takes its place, because man always directs his efforts toward some good or other. Thus utility becomes something which the intelligence is no longer entitled to define or to judge, but only to serve" (Weil, 1968, p. 63).

THE RELIGION FACTOR

Although scholars and researchers for centuries have attempted to formulate a clear definition of religion, none has surfaced. However, there have been responsible and serious attempts, particularly by religious scholars who have established a monumental reservoir of work. Perhaps one of the most influential scholars of religion is the American Huston Smith (1991). Smith writes that "authentic religion is the clearest opening through which the inexhaustible energies of the cosmos enter our lives. . . . (p. 9). Taken in its widest sense, [it is] a way of life woven around a people's ultimate concern . . . in its narrower sense [it is] a concern to align humanity with the transcendental ground of its being" (p. 183). The scientific community–at least that splinter of it represented in health care–has taken such a profound understanding of religion and decided to call it "spirituality"; and in the process has endeavored to dilute religion to only one of its forms–institutional religion.

Given the hostility between science and religion over the centuries, such an intellectual trick is understandable. What is less comprehensible is that chaplaincy–an expression of a religious ministry–would not hold the scientific community to a more responsible project of scholarship and historic sensitivity.

Much of this argument, I realize, may be dismissed with the shibboleths of "postmodernism" or "practicality" in the face of political and financial forces, but surely the education of religious professionals, including the inclusion of a powerful prophetic dimension, would dictate a more enlightened and vigorous resistance to the sundry attempts to delegate religion to a sub-system within spirituality.

Even if one comes down hard on the argument that clinical pastoral education and professional chaplaincy need to be "more scientific," such a conversion of meaning is hardly defensible, for, as already noted, most scientific research demonstrates a possible link between religion and health, not spirituality and health.

Indeed, this body of research provides an excellent illustration of how scientism, the exaggerated worship of science and scientific method, may restrict and distort the notion of religion. It is important to note in this regard that the issue being discussed–that is, should chaplaincy become more scientific in response to health care reform–often made manifest in the area of research methodology.

Since the beginnings of the pastoral care and counseling movement, there has been a persistent complaint regarding the movement's lack of research (Strunk, 1998). A close examination of this body of literature reveals, however, that the lament is not focused so much on a paucity of research but rather on a lack of *quantitative* research. Often, the critics are informed or driven by a chain of unexamined "givens"; namely, science's roots in the philosophy of logical positivism and its primary methodology and epistemology of empiricism. Although these philosophical positions are rarely challenged, or even recognized, by contemporary enthusiasts of quantitative research, in this new century and in the last half of the last century–particularly with the rise of the human sciences (as contrasted to the physical sciences)–a strictly quantitative dogma has come under critical analysis. Indeed, it has been cogently argued that many of the issues facing caregivers, including chaplains, pastoral counselors, and pastoral educators, might better be addressed by carefully designing and carrying out qualitative approaches to perplexing issues frequently faced by chaplains (O'Connor, 2001).

Also, often overlooked in this lively discourse is the reality that within religion itself there exists a lengthy and intense research tradition, a form one active pastoral care researcher has termed *heuristic* research (Thomas St. John O'Connor, personal communication, December 05, 2001). This reality should hint that science–or perhaps a misunderstanding of authentic science–cannot provide professional chaplaincy with a sufficient foundation for its mission and that its role might better be considered as an important but nevertheless an auxiliary one, along with other areas of inquiry.

CHAPLAINCY

By this time the reader will recognize that much of what has been argued in this response will be valued or disvalued by how one conceives the identity and role of professional chaplaincy in the health care project. And here I can only offer a perspective based partly on my understanding of the history of CPE and chaplaincy and partly on what appears to me evident in the *Zeitgeist;* namely, that pastoral caregivers today, whether chaplains or pastoral counselor, are called to be radically systemic in their expressions of ministry (Strunk, 1995).

By history and calling, the chaplaincy of the future cannot afford to stand within a tight, narrow, limiting circle of meaning. The contemporary chaplain will need to take seriously the notion that *religion*, which chaplains represent, is indeed a "universal entity that, as indicated by its etymology, somehow binds things back to itself" (Leeming, 2001, p. 115). Religion is, as Huston Smith has noted, ". . . a way of life woven around a people's ultimate concern . . ."

What this means in regard to the central concern of this response is that chaplaincy, born as it was as a "sector ministry" (Legood, 1989), has a responsibility to draw as much as possible on authentic science (not scientism) but ought never allow itself to be limited or in any sense intimidated by that particular world. Instead, the chaplain needs to strive to be what William James called the "complete philosopher"–the person who is required to be aware and sensitive to many sub-universes and to determine the relations of those sub-universes at the moment of critical need.

The chaplain and the CPE educator are constantly challenged to recognize that all systemic forces are most evident and realistically addressed as they are concentralized in persons with whom chaplains are called to serve (Strunk, 1995). To this ideal end, chaplains will surely need all the resources and methods available from science, art, the humanities, literature, theology, ethics, and religious studies.

REFERENCES

Allport, G. W. (1937). *Personality: A psychological interpretation.* New York: Henry Holt & Co.

Frost, C., & Bell-Metereau, R. (1998). *Simone Weil: On politics, religion, and society.* London: SAGE Publications, Ltd.

Hall, C. E. (1992). *Head and heart: The story of the clinical pastoral education movement.* Decatur, GA: Journal of Pastoral Care Publications, Inc.

James, W. (1890). *The principles of psychology.* New York: Henry Holt.

Koenig, H. G., McCullough, M. E., & Larson, D. B. (2001). *Handbook on religion and health.* Oxford: Oxford University Press.

Koenig, H. G. (1997). *Is religion good for your health? Effects of religion on mental and physical health.* New York: The Haworth Press, Inc.

Larson, D. B., Swyers, J. P., & McCullough, M. E. (1998). *Scientific research on spirituality and health: A consensus report.* Rockville, MD: National Institute for Healthcare Research.

Leeming, D. A. (2001). Myth and therapy. *Journal of Religion and Health, 40,* 1, 115-119.

Legood, G. (1999). *Chaplaincy: The church's sector ministries.* London: Cassell.

Means, J. J. (2002). Mighty prophet/wounded healer. *The Journal of Pastoral Care & Counseling* (in press).

O'Connor, T. S. J., Meaks, E., Davis, K., Koning, F., McLernon-Sinclair, K., & Vanessa, L. (2001). Quantity and rigor of qualitative research in four pastoral counseling journals. *The Journal of Pastoral Care, 55,* 271-280.

Smith, H. (1991). *The world's religions* (rev. ed). New York: HarperCollins.

Strunk, O., Jr. (1995). Multicultural counseling and the systemic notion: Implications for pastoral psychotherapy. In Carole R. Bohn (Ed.), *Therapeutic practice in a cross-cultural world: Theological, psychological, and ethical issues.* (pp. 3-15). Decatur, GA: Journal of Pastoral Care Publications, Inc.

Strunk, O., Jr. (1990). Research in the pastoral arts and sciences: A reassessment. *Journal of Pastoral Psychotherapy, 21,* 3-12.

VandeCreek, L., & Burton, L. (Eds.) (2001). Professional chaplaincy: Its role and importance in healthcare. *The Journal of Pastoral Care, 55,* 81-97.

Weaver, A. J., Koenig, H. G., & Roe, P. C. (1998). *Reflections on aging and spiritual growth.* Nashville: Abingdon Press.

Weil, S. (1968). *On science, necessity, and the love of God.* London: Oxford University Press.

Rediscovering Mystery and Wonder: Toward a Narrative-Based Perspective on Chaplaincy

Rev. Dr. John Swinton, PhD, BD, RMN, RNMH

SUMMARY. Should chaplaincy be scientific? The answer is a resounding yes! Science is not the enemy of chaplaincy any more than it is the enemy of theology. It is necessary and therapeutically vital that chaplains strive to base their theory and practice on appropriate and well-researched evidence. The substantial question, however, is: What actually constitutes acceptable evidence, who decides and why? *[Article copies available for a fee from The Haworth Document Delivery Service: 1-800-HAWORTH. E-mail address: <docdelivery@haworthpress.com> Website: <http://www.HaworthPress.com> © 2002 by The Haworth Press, Inc. All rights reserved.]*

KEYWORDS. Chaplaincy, religion, science, research

Rev. Dr. John Swinton is Senior Lecturer in Practical Theology, School of Divinity and Religious Studies, King's College, University of Aberdeen, Aberdeen, Scotland (E-mail: j.swinton@abdn.ac.uk).

The author is indebted to colleague Mark Cobb who is a Senior Chaplain at the Sheffield University Teaching Hospitals NHS Trust, Sheffield, England, UK. It was he whom the author first heard using the metaphor of the waterfall in relation to human spirituality.

[Haworth co-indexing entry note]: "Rediscovering Mystery and Wonder: Toward a Narrative-Based Perspective on Chaplaincy." Swinton, John. Co-published simultaneously in *Journal of Health Care Chaplaincy* (The Haworth Social Work Practice Press, an imprint of The Haworth Press, Inc.) Vol. 13, No. 1, 2002, pp. 223-236; and: *Professional Chaplaincy and Clinical Pastoral Education Should Become More Scientific: Yes and No* (ed: Larry VandeCreek) The Haworth Pastoral Press, an imprint of The Haworth Press, Inc., 2003, pp. 223-236. Single or multiple copies of this article are available for a fee from The Haworth Document Delivery Service [1-800-HAWORTH, 9:00 a.m. - 5:00 p.m. (EST). E-mail address: docdelivery@haworthpress.com].

10.1300/J080v13n01_06

Imagine yourself walking through a deep, dense wood. You are surrounded by beautiful, luscious foliage; the constantly changing aromas of the rich shrubbery makes your head swirl. Suddenly you reach a clearing. Right in the centre of the clearing is a beautiful stream headed up by a magnificence waterfall. You stand and watch in awe at the mystery and wonder of the waterfall. Multiple rainbows dance across the glistening surface of the water. The sound of the water, the taste of the spray, the sight of the magnificence and power of the waterfall touches you in inexpressible places and brings you into contact with a dimension of experience which you can't quite articulate, but which you feel deeply and meaningfully. Eventually, your gaze of wonder begins to change as your curious side clicks into action: "What is this thing called a waterfall?" "What is it made of?" "Why does it have such an effect on me?" So, you pick up a bucket and scoop up some of the water from the falls. You look into the bucket, but something has changed. The water is of course technically the same substance in each setting: H_2O. It remains a vital constituent in your life; you need it to live and without it you will perish. Yet, something has been lost in the movement from waterfall to bucket. In your attempts to break it down, analyse and explain what it really is, the mystery and awe of the waterfall has been left behind. Which is more real: The mystery of the crashing waterfall or the still waters of the bucket?

I think this word picture reveals an important dimension that sits at the heart of the current debate over the role of the chaplain within a professional, evidence based, scientifically driven healthcare system. On the one hand, chaplains are called to be spiritual healers and carers. They are called to mediate and care for a person's spirituality: that dimension of humanness that is unquantifiable, mysterious, individual and unique. On the other hand, they are called to justify their existence within a healthcare context that places great emphasis on that which is quantifiable, generalizable and universally applicable. The tension between the waterfall and the still waters of the bucket symbolises the difficult tension that chaplains are faced with when they begin to consider their role the healthcare system. In terms of professional development and their long-term role within the healthcare system this tension requires to be reflected on sensitively and thoughtfully in order that the uniqueness of chaplaincy can be fully recognised and effectively and meaningfully worked out.

SHOULD CHAPLAINCY BE SCIENTIFIC?

The answer to this question is a resounding yes! Science is not the enemy of chaplaincy any more than it is the enemy of theology. Chaplains are called to provide the best, most appropriate care possible. It is right and proper that they should be aware of scientific developments and be able to function effectively within an environment whose primary language is often scientific. Chaplaincy is correct to utilise the methodologies of science to explore and reveal dimensions of its own practice that will enable chaplains to function more effectively and to care more fully. Chaplaincy needs to be evidence based and the very real and important contribution that chaplains make needs to be brought clearly to the attention of managers, administrators, fellow professionals and patients alike in order that this dimension of healthcare can be recognised, valued and developed in ways which are constructive and health-bringing. It is necessary and therapeutically vital that chaplains strive to base their theory and practice on appropriate and well-researched evidence.

However, the question is: What actually constitutes acceptable evidence, who decides and why? The easy option is for chaplaincy simply to hang on the coat tails of medical science and technology and try to establish itself as a 'professional' discipline using the particular criterion of professionalism that are deemed to be legitimate at this moment in time. Currently it is the so-called 'hard sciences' that are assumed to provide the plausibility structures for sound, evidence based professional practice within the healthcare arena. When we talk about adopting evidence based, scientific approach to chaplaincy we tend to assume a very narrow understanding of science and ways in which we can authentically attain meaningful human knowledge. For knowledge to be deemed 'truth' it must be tangible, scientifically verifiable and consequently generalizable and reproducible.

However, I suggest that science, or at least a narrow definition of science, is only one dimension of the professional role of chaplaincy. On its own our current definition of 'science' cannot provide an adequate basis for the theory and practice of chaplaincy. Why? Because human beings in general and human spirituality in particular is more akin to a waterfall than to the still waters of a bucket. Chaplains are first and foremost called to care for the spirituality of human beings, i.e., that dimension of humanness that refuses to be captured by standard scientific methods. If chaplains in their quest for 'professional credibility' forget this, they risk losing something that is fundamental to authentic chaplaincy.

PSYCHOLOGICAL MODERNISM

As I reflect on the nature of some dimensions of the discussion on whether or not chaplains should become more scientific in their approach, I get uneasy. Not because I have a problem with science. My uneasiness is caused by some underlying assumptions that, in the long term, may prove to be counterproductive and perhaps even dangerous. Thomas Moore has described a condition he calls psychological modernism: an uncritical acceptance of the values and understandings that make up the worldview of the modern world (Moore 1993). Such a view restricts the parameters within which decisions are made, situations are assessed and understood and persons are treated, to the idea that the practice of healthcare can progress towards the freedom from illness and distress through the accumulation of human knowledge using the methodologies of empiricism and statistical quantifiability as the ultimate criterion for the development of identity and professional credibility. So called 'soft knowledge' like spirituality sits very uneasily within this modernist mindset. Spirituality is not easily quantified by scientific methodologies and assumptions; its manifestations are often unique and non-generalizable, and its central tenets of love, relationship, hope transcendence and meaning, are not easily fitted into auditable competences. Psychological modernism leaves little room for those less quantifiable aspects of care. Instead as Moore correctly points out, 'technology' rather than 'theology' becomes the root metaphor for dealing with health and illness (Moore 1993).

Such implicit or explicit psychological modernism is one of the main dangers that any narrow turn by chaplaincy towards science could bring about. While scientific knowledge is necessary, in its narrow positivistic form, it is certainly not sufficient for developing an understanding of the professional role of the chaplain. It simply does not provide a sufficient basis for developing a meaningful understanding of what it means to be human and to live humanly in the midst of disease and suffering. The danger for all of us who work within a contemporary healthcare context is that in our quest for professional/scientific credibility and our growing dependence on physical and psychological technology, we forget what it means to be human and to live humanly. Chaplaincy cannot afford to take that chance. If, even implicitly, it loses sight of the fullness of human beings and locks itself into a one-dimensional approach that does little justice to the richness and diversity that is a primary mark of human existence, chaplaincy will have failed in a fundamental way. Statistics, numbers and randomised control trials can offer us some knowledge of human beings and human experience, but on there own these dimensions of science cannot capture the "awesomeness of the waterfall." If chaplains are to take seriously the ideas of science and evidence based practice, I would suggest that they must expand their definitions of what science is and what constitutes legitimate evidence, to include those dimensions of human experience which make human living human. This being so, any meaningful discussion of a scientific basis for chaplaincy must begin with the premise that the fundamental task of chaplaincy is not simply to conform to current professional standards but also to transform them in ways which reflect and cater for the fullness of human beings and the rich diversity of human spiritual experience.

REDISCOVERING MYSTERY AND WONDER: DEVELOPING AN EXPANDED SCIENCE

Chaplains are called to rediscover the mystery and wonder of the waterfalls. Whilst many dimensions of scientifically based healthcare begin with the assumption of that which can be captured and analyzed "in a bucket" will reveal the "true" nature of the thing being examined, the chaplain is called to widen that understanding to incorporate the dimensions of being human which often fall outside the standard medical gaze. In the words of William James,

Many worlds of consciousness exist . . . which have a meaning for our life . . . the total expression of human experience . . . invincibly urges me beyond the narrow "scientific" bounds. Assuredly, the real world is of different temperament–more intricately built than physical science allows. (William James in Richard and Bergin 1997, p. 21)

The task of chaplaincy is to explore and mediate these other worlds and to enable other healthcare professionals to begin to expand their vision of science and the meaning of healing, wholeness and humanness. Chaplaincy is called to consider the possibility of developing what Abraham Maslow (1985) has neatly defined as an 'expanded science'; a form of science which takes seriously issues of value, hope, meaning and the unpredictable nature of lived experience. Such an approach will not exclude scientific methodology or the standard methods of science that have undoubtedly brought much benefit and healing. However, it will seek to explore the possibility that chaplaincy might have a unique, if often overlooked dimension which it can add to the theory and practice of healthcare; a dimension which may not be available to any other discipline, but which is vital for truly holistic healthcare.

NARRATIVE BASED CHAPLAINCY

Within nursing and medicine, as well as various disciplines in the social sciences such as psychology and sociology, there has recently been a significant movement towards the therapeutic significance of narrative for understandings of health and illness. The work of clinicians such as Arthur Kleinman (1988), Oliver Sacks (1998), and Richard Seltzer (2002) have opened up the significance of illness narratives, not simply as illustration to confirm or disconfirm diagnostic assumptions, but as a unique media which reveal new or "forgotten" dimensions of health and illness. In listening to the stories of those to whom we seek to offer care, we are confronted with new realities, embodied spiritual truths and deep and meaningful insights into the experience of illness and the implications of this for genuinely person-centred care. In a techno-medical (Wigg 1995 in Nolan and Crawford 1997) context that may well have forgotten what it means to be human and to live humanly, such a revelation is crucial. I want to propose that it is within the realm of narrative that chaplaincy can find a sure foundation for its theory and professional practice. Narrative offers a conduit through which chaplains can make a genuine and unique contribution to the development of healthcare practices and offer vital insights and new competencies to the healthcare team.

TAKING STORIES SERIOUSLY

Before we can begin to take narrative seriously, it is necessary to think through what narrative actually is and the ways in which it functions in human life. Put simply, stories are "the linguistic form most related to the way people maintain a sense of continuity through time and a primary form in which they share experience" (Ruffing 1989 p. 62). A person's story reveals not only what they do or what they have, it also reveals who they are and how they perceive themselves to be. A person's story reveals the way they construct the universe and their place within it. Stories reveal more than symptoms and diagnoses. They reveal the particular meaning and purpose a person's illness has for them. This story may differ from the one told about the patient by the healthcare professional. It may be subsumed or subordinated to the medical discourse that often reigns omnipotent. However, when listened to, such stories can be a rich source of spiritual revelation and therapeutic healing. Whilst issues of meaning and purpose might not be considered central to the standard methods of science, when it comes to dealing with real people in real life situations, this dimension is crucial.

Human beings are by nature storytellers. "We work and worry, pray and play, love and hate; and all the time we are telling stories about our pasts, our presents and our futures . . . everywhere we go, we are charged with telling stories and making meaning–giving sense to ourselves and the world around us (Plummer 1995 p. 20). When we seek to make sense of our experiences, including our experience of illness we fit them into stories." When events fall into a pattern which we can describe in a way that is satisfying as narrative then we think that we have some grasp of why they occurred. (Dictionary of philosophy p. 853). In *The Man Who Mistook His Wife for a Hat* Oliver Sacks puts this point thus:

> If we wish to know a man, we ask, 'what is his story, his real, inmost story?' For each of us is a biography, a story. Each of us is a singular narrative, which is constructed continually and unconsciously by, through, and in us–through our perceptions, our feelings, our thoughts, our actions; and, not least, through our discourse, our spoken narrations. Biologically, physiologically, we are not so different from each other; historically, as narratives, we are each of us unique. (Sacks p. 1988).

It is our narrative experience that provides us with our uniqueness and individuality. While we may have dimensions of our selves and our experiences that are quantifiable, reproducible and generalizable, our personal narratives, like our spirituality, provide a dimension of our experience that is unique, ungeneralizable and unrepeatable. As such a person's story holds the potential to reveal unique dimensions of illness experience unavailable by other means.

Bearing in mind the increasing emphasis on technology within the practice of healthcare, this is no small point. As Greenhaugh points out, At its most arid, modern medicine lacks a metric for existential qualities such as the inner hurt, despair, hope, grief, and moral pain that frequently accompany and often indeed constitute, the illness from which people suffer. (Greenhaugh 1999 quoting from Balint 1957 p. 50)

If Greenhaugh is correct in this assertion, it has important implications for chaplaincy. The existential/spiritual dimensions of the healthcare process that are highlighted by Greenhaugh as missing from contemporary healthcare practices form the very essence of chaplaincy. It is in recognising and seeking to offer care and insight into these dimension that chaplaincy consolidates its unique position within the healthcare system Rather than simply attempting to latch on to a research agenda which is frequently set within a narrowly scientific model which excludes vital dimensions of humanness, a focus which seeks to reflect critically on people's stories and which exposes the hidden existential dimensions of health and illness will enable chaplains to add a vital and often missing dimension to the contemporary understanding and practice of healthcare.

THE CHAPLAINS THE BEARER AND SHARER OF STORIES

On reflection, such an emphasis for professional chaplaincy seems rather obvious. If we think for a moment on the day-to-day practice of chaplaincy, it becomes clear that the idea of narrative is central to the role of the chaplain. Religious communities are formed around particular sets of narratives which present varying interpretations of what life is about, who God is and what it means to be human and to live humanly. Such communities tell stories about health, illness, sadness and joy and offer explanatory narratives within which people can make sense of their lives. Particular religious communities normally commission chaplains. They are sent out by religious communities and charged with the responsibility of embodying, acting out and, where appropriate, re-telling in healing ways, the particular narrative of their religious communities. All day-long they tell and listen to stories, stories of illness, sickness, suffering, happiness, brokenness, life and death. This storied universe provides the basic context for chaplaincy and represents a primary mode of communication and healing that they offer to those with whom they come into contact. This being so, surely, in terms of establishing a professional role for chaplains, it is this dimension of human experience that provides chaplaincy with a particular dynamic and a distinctive focus?

LISTENING TO STORIES AND RECREATING WORLDS

Stories then are the mode through which people make sense of their world and their experiences within that world. As such, interpreting people's stories holds the potential to provide deep insights into the nature and meaning of illness and illness experiences. It is my proposition that the role of chaplaincy in expanding science and moving healthcare practices from the stillness of the bucket to wonder of the waterfall can be consolidated by developing the concept and significance of narrative and introducing a hermeneutical/interpretative dimension to its research and practice. An illustration from my own research will help make my point.

LIVING WITH SADNESS: THE LIVED EXPERIENCE OF DEPRESSION

The project I will highlight focussed on the lived experience of spirituality within the context of long-term depression. The full report of the study can be read elsewhere (Swinton 2001). Here I will explore a section of the report. It drew upon a hermeneutical-phenomenological qualitative methodology and sought to develop deep and meaningful understandings of what depression is as a human experience rather than simply a diagnostic category.

CROSSING OVER INTO STRANGE LANDS

The study drew together methodological concepts from the philosopher Hans Georg Gadamer (Gadamer 1981) and the thinking of the pastoral theologian David Augsberger (Augsberger 1986) in order to explore some dynamics of narrative and its implications for our understanding of the spiritual dynamics of depression. Augsberger, in his work on cross-cultural counselling, develops the concept of interpathy. Interpathy relates to the researcher or a practitioner crossing over into a culture that is radically different from their own. It requires that the person temporarily suspend their assumptions about the world and how it should function and take on board fully the reality of the world as perceived by those who dwell in the different culture. This idea relates well with the suggestion that narratives can reveal hidden truths. If we take the concept of interpathy into a healthcare context it can provide a useful tool of exploration and understanding. Susan Sontag describes the worlds of health and illness as two different countries (Sontag 1991). With that analogy in mind, in like-manner to crossing over into a different culture, entering the worlds of ill people can be compared with entering into strange new lands; new lands within which the world can look very different. In these "strange places," our standard understandings of reality and normality are challenged and reshaped as we listen to the stories told by those who unwillingly dwell there. Adopting the concept of interpathy as a critical tool of excavation, designed to enable chaplains to research and practice authentically and effectively, requires a revised mindset that moves beyond scientific methods and dislocated diagnostic assumptions and enables the chaplain genuinely to enter into the "foreign country" of illness, to sit down and to look around. It relates to chaplains learning skills of spiritual exploration that will allow them, as far as is possible, to enter into the spiritual experience of the sick person and feel comfortable sitting in those realms that are not part of the normal therapeutic world. To enter interpathically into the situation of an ill person means entering into their experience with more than science, diagnostic categories and therapeutic techniques at our fingertips. It requires that the chaplain takes the experience of the patient with the utmost seriousness and attempts to understand what that experience is like and what it means to the person "from the inside."

UNDERSTANDING SADNESS

The research discussed here involved a number of in-depth interviews with people who have experienced depression over an extended period of time. The objective was not to explain depression, but to seek to understand it. In seeking to understand depression, it was hoped that fresh insights might arise which would lead to improved strategies and more empathetic caring practices. The following excerpt from the narrative of one woman who suffers from enduring depression will show the revelatory power of this approach. In this abstract the woman is describing the significance of meaning for her life and reflecting on the ways in which depression destroys her sense of meaning and purpose:

> I don't depend on there being direct, individual meaning in my particular circumstances or situation and all the bad things that happen to me. I'm quite happy to live with the idea that, you know, in a fallen world there are things that happen to people just sort of through

chance and circumstance. But what one does need to believe is that all of that is happening in an ultimately meaningful framework.

However, if that ultimately meaningful framework collapses, as is the case when she tumbles into the depths of depression, she is catapulted into a deep dark void that is deeply disturbing and spiritually devastating. She describes this experience as "an abyss."

> When I'm in a phase that I am able to believe that there is a God who gives meaning to that universe, then I have hope. But there have been spells when I haven't been able to believe that, and that has been absolutely terrifying. That's been falling into the abyss. That is seriously nasty!

The imagery of the abyss powerfully symbolizes the terrifying black pit of meaninglessness into which a person slides during the experience of depression. The only foothold out of the abyss is the possibility that there is meaning beyond one's own situation. If this foothold is torn away, there is "nothing but 'nothingness' and darkness."

> You would go to bed at night and it was dark outside, and it felt dark inside. All creative energy was gone, it just wasn't there. When I woke in the morning, although it was dawn, inside nothing had changed and it was still dark.

The abyss is filled with doubt about self, others and the order of the world. It is a meaningless void within which strength, hope and light are drained, leaving the person in a dark and lonely place.

What is perhaps worse is the fact that those who have to live with the threat of depression on a long time basis are faced with the possibility of living under the shadow of the abyss for all time.

> Even when I am well its like I am always wandering around the edge of the abyss, always looking over the edge, knowing that at any time I could slip and plunge back in. . . . that is not a good way to live your life.

Viewed through the eyes of the persons story

> The idea of suicide is the most rational thing in the world when you are going through all that pain. It's the people who try to stop

you that you think are off their heads. Why would you want to go on living if you felt like that?

While a strictly biomedical perspective might simply write off suicide as irrational behavior, a narrative-hermeneutical perspective reveals it as a rational response to a particularly unpleasant human experience. What is required in terms of a therapeutic response is not simply medication, but also deep understanding, what I would describe as *therapeutic understanding*. Such understanding breaks down the isolation of the experience and opens up the possibility of offering alternative ways of viewing and caring for the individual's situation. As one woman put it:

> You don't have to believe what I believe to give me spiritual care, but you have to have empathy and the understanding that this person requires this . . . its part of her . . . [carers need to be able to say] "I may not believe it but because she needs it then we'll try and provide that for her."

Research such as this is both rigorous and scientific (Sandelowski 1986), yet it draws us beyond the boundaries of techno-medicine and reintroduces the fullness of the person to the process of healthcare. In so doing chaplains who choose to utilise this approach, can enable clinicians to develop deep insights into the depths of human experience and in so doing, enable all to ask different questions which in turn will lead to more effective healthcare practices. In asking different questions we can begin to see and to understand the world of illness differently and be opened up to new ways of caring, healing and 'being with' the sick. Drawing the attention of healthcare professionals to this vital narrative dimension of human experience is a major contribution that chaplains can offer to others within the multidisciplinary healthcare team.

IS STORYTELLING RESEARCH?

The answer to this is certainly yes! But it is based on an understanding of science that is broader than that which we might normally assume. Doing interpretative research based on listening to and reflecting on stories is not an easy option. It is rigorous, based on sound methodologies and designed to increase human knowledge and understanding (Koch 1998). As such it provides possibilities for an expanded scientific approach that is different from but complimentary to standard scientific approaches. There are of course philosophical and methodological differences between this approach and that of mainline science (Lincoln and Guba 1985). However, these differences should be treated as acting in a complementary fashion to reveal different but harmonious aspects of the experience of illness and the practice of healthcare.

'EITHER OR' OR 'BOTH AND'?

To suggest a narrative based approach to the theory and practice of chaplaincy is not to suggest that chaplains should ignore standard scientific methods. As I have tried to make clear, science should be seen as complementary rather than antipathetic to a narrative based model of chaplaincy. However, chaplains are not primarily scientists, at least not in the way in which we have come to conceive that term. They are first and foremost spiritual carers, charged with the responsibility of revealing the therapeutic significance of those dimensions of human experience that are mysterious and wonderful. At least part of this task relates to the chaplain's ability to enable the healing knowledge of the patient's story to find a voice amidst the cacophony of disparate voices that pervade the healthcare system.

Chaplains have a unique and vital contribution to make to the practice of healthcare. However, they will only effectively make that contribution if they are prepared to take the chance of holding onto that which is unique to chaplaincy. If they simply follow on behind the other healthcare disciplines and try to do the same things in the same ways, they will lose their healing and transforming power. Chaplains must be brave enough to grasp the significance and uniqueness of their own discipline, even if this means failing to establish themselves on the basis that appears strongest at this moment in time. Rather than becoming "scientific" in the narrow, positivistic way that many other disciplines interpret and work out this word, chaplains need to reflect seriously on the possibility of expanding current understandings of science to include those dimensions of spirituality and humanness which are often hidden in the midst of a techno-medical system which seems at times to worship scientific methodology at the expense of that which makes human living human. Chaplains are not called to conform to that which is assumed to be most credible. Rather, their calling is to enable healthy transformation at a personal and a systemic level by revealing hidden spiritual dynamics which may not be measurable or repeatable, but which provide the very fabric of meaningful human existence. Chaplains must begin to draw people's gaze away from the stillness of the water in the bucket back towards the mystery and wonder of the waterfall. In doing that they will be offering contemporary healthcare practices something beautiful and deeply needed.

REFERENCES

Augsberger, D. W. (1986). *Pastoral Counselling Across Cultures.* Philadelphia: Westminster Press.

Balint, M. (1957). *The doctor, his patient and the illness.* London: Tavistock Publications.

Gadamer, Hans-Georg. (1981). *Truth and Method.* London: Sheed and Ward.

Greenhalgh, Trisha and Hurwitz, Brian. (1999). 'Narrative based medicine: Why study narrative?' *British Medical Journal, http://bmj.com.*

Honderich, Ted (ed.). (1995). *The Oxford Companion to Philosophy.* New York: Oxford University Press.

Kleinman, Arthur. (1988). *The Illness Narratives: Suffering, Healing & The Human Condition.* Basic Books, United States of America.

Koch, Tina. (1998). 'Story telling: Is it really research.' *Journal of Advanced Nursing.* 28(6): 118-1190.

Lincoln, Yvonna S., and Guba, Egon G. (1985). *Naturalistic Enquiry.* London: Sage Publications.

Maslow, A. (1985). *The Farther Reaches of Human Nature.* New York: Penguin.

Moore, Thomas. (1992). *Care of the Soul: A Guide for Cultivating Depth and Sacredness in Everyday Live.* New York: HarperCollins.

Nolan P. and Crawford P. (1997). Towards a rhetoric of spirituality in mental health care. *Journal of Advanced Nursing.* 26(2): 289-94.

Plummer, Ken. (1985). *Telling Sexual Stories: Power, Change and Social Worlds.* Routledge, London and New York.

Richards, P. Scott and Bergin, Allen E. (1997). *A Spiritual Strategy for Counselling and Psychotherapy.* American Psychological Association, Washington.

Ruffing, Janet. (1989). *Uncovering Stories of Faith.* NY: Paulist Press.

Sacks, Oliver. (1998). *The Man Who Mistook His Wife for a Hat.* Touchstone Books.

Sandelowski, M. (1986). The problem of rigour in qualitative research. *Advances in Nursing Science,* 8, 3: 27-37.

Selzer, Richard. (2002). *The Exact Location of the Soul.* Picador USA.

Sontag, Susan. (1991). *Illness As Metaphor Aids and its Metaphors.* Penguin Books, London.

Wigg, N. N. (1995). Plenary Lecture Delivered at the Mary Hemingway Rees Memorial Lecture. World Federation of Mental Health, Trinity College, Dublin, August.

Attention to the Scientific Benefits
of Pastoral Care Is a Blessing and a Curse

The Reverend Jo Clare Wilson, MDiv

SUMMARY. The art of pastoral care may be difficult to describe but we know that the ability to measure and describe the process of becoming a clinically trained, professional pastoral care provider is possible. Within the Association for Clinical Pastoral Education we have developed standards that spell out the competencies needed to complete the desired skill outcomes. Instead of diluting the meaning of pastoral care, this movement has strengthened the training, at least for many supervisors, students and seminaries. I argue that being able to understand with more precision what we do and how we do it could only enhance the practice of our art and the understanding by others of what that art might look like. *[Article copies available for a fee from The Haworth Document Delivery Service: 1-800-HAWORTH. E-mail address: <docdelivery@haworthpress.com> Website: <http://www.HaworthPress.com> © 2002 by The Haworth Press, Inc. All rights reserved.]*

KEYWORDS. Chaplaincy, clinical pastoral education, science, research

---

The Reverend Jo Clare Wilson is affiliated with The Healthcare Chaplaincy, Inc., and Director, Pastoral Care and Education, Griffin Hospital, Derby, CT 06418 (E-mail: grifpc@griffinhealth.org).

[Haworth co-indexing entry note]: "Attention to the Scientific Benefits of Pastoral Care Is a Blessing and a Curse." Wilson, Jo Clare. Co-published simultaneously in *Journal of Health Care Chaplaincy* (The Haworth Pastoral Press, an imprint of The Haworth Press, Inc.) Vol. 13, No. 1, 2002, pp. 237-244; and: *Professional Chaplaincy and Clinical Pastoral Education Should Become More Scientific: Yes and No* (ed: Larry VandeCreek) The Haworth Pastoral Press, an imprint of The Haworth Press, Inc., 2003, pp. 237-244. Single or multiple copies of this article are available for a fee from The Haworth Document Delivery Service [1-800-HAWORTH, 9:00 a.m. - 5:00 p.m. (EST). E-mail address: docdelivery@haworthpress.com].

10.1300/J080v13n01_07   *237*

For the last several years I have become increasingly encouraged as I hear more concerning the enlightened discovery made by physicians, nurses and allied health care professionals about how spirituality impacts the reality of disease and wellness. Yet, I have also become increasingly dismayed, as I continue to hear more about the enlightened "discovery" made by physicians, nurses and allied health care professionals about how spirituality impacts the reality of disease and wellness.

When asked to respond to the question, "Should clinical pastoral education and professional chaplaincy become more scientific in response to health care reform?" my response is ambivalence. This "new" attention to the scientific benefits of pastoral care is a blessing and a curse.

I believe most of us in professional chaplaincy are struggling with the current surge of research, which seems to support and undermine us at the same time. This phenomenon also taps into our resistance and authority. (Of course I would name those two as pertinent issues as an aging CPE supervisor; after all don't we see resistance and authority "issues" in everything?)

Obviously the support and encouragement being felt among the pastoral care community stems from having other disciplines recognize what most of us have worked with and known for generations, i.e., the effects of a healthy faith upon the healing process. The medical practitioners who are recognizing the contributions of pastoral care are higher up in the pecking order (physicians, nurses and scientists) as well as being indispensable in the medical world. Chaplains, we know all too well, are dispensable. Hence, our authority issues.

The sense of being undermined happens when we encounter those who would either overtly or covertly require that we give empirical *proof* that what we practice is actually worth the money. I have participated in countless meetings that push Chaplains and Spiritual caregivers to increase patient satisfaction scores in the area of "spiritual and emotional needs " (Press-Ganey is the most pervasive example). I have found myself reaching to do all sorts of marketing techniques to ensure that those needs are met, for example, creating printed signs, brochures, tray cards, etc. about pastoral services to distribute in each room. I have instructed volunteers and CPE students see *every patient* in order that there is an increased awareness of spiritual care. I have seen staff wearing pins and buttons with the slogans "strive for five" and "ask me what that means." This is done as a means to help patients know for certain that we will be asking them to give us high marks in that patient satisfaction spiritual score. These efforts only increase my resistance.

I do teach nurses how to do a "spiritual assessment" in order that patients are referred properly. The latter has always been a portion of what I believe to be a solid pastoral care strategy since we depend on referrals and it does increase the awareness of the effects of spiritual issues on health. But I can also become defensive and a bit reactionary when the push begins to include remarks that indicate nurses should be doing spiritual care and I should be designing courses to provide such education.

Don't get me wrong. It is my opinion that spiritual care is a part of the whole care of the patient and many wonderful nurses I have worked with through the years include spirituality in their practice. Therefore it is important to discuss the difference between what a nurse might do as a spiritual care and when to call for the chaplain. Sometimes I feel as though I go back and forth between excitements at spiritual needs being recognized and fear that perhaps the role of Chaplain may someday be obsolete. This also leads to resistance.

A somewhat aside observation that could perhaps be another study for research involves the difference I have experienced between chaplaincy in the North and in the South. In the South, I worried at times that my "territory" was being infringed upon when some nurses prayed with patients and then began evangelizing. There was at least one person per week who asked another chaplain or myself how they, too, could be a chaplain. They were always surprised that a person actually needed training. For many southern religious folks who happened to be nurses there was the thought that anyone who felt "called by the Lord" could do the task.

In the North, in contrast, I have observed how many people have not a clue about what chaplains might do and are more distant and uncertain about the part that religion plays in patient care. What often happens in this scenario is that there is a rush to embrace "spirituality," since this more ambiguous term is perceived as less religious and perhaps less threatening. As spirituality becomes more pervasive the inclination may be to dilute the religious, institutional and communal nature of chaplaincy. So resistance contains underneath the anger at having to prove and define what I do in order to gain and maintain professional recognition and respect.

I present three themes as my contribution to this discussion. The first theme concerns the nature and function of science as it pertains to both health care and theology. Should we be asked to "prove" our worth by becoming more scientific?

My second theme touches on the art of pastoral care. Will a more scientific approach change our understanding so that the art of pastoral care will be lost in the rush to examine and define the discipline? Might this fear represent an assumption (whether spoken or unspoken) that by defining and measuring we are destroying the "sacred" nature of our work? Is pastoral care exempt from scrutiny because the very nature of the discipline evolves around a mystery of faith that I believe can be found in most all religious traditions? This assumption would equate the process of defining and empirically proving the effects of pastoral care with a loss of power and respect.

Finally, I claim that a professional and responsible response will not opt for the scientific over the sacred or vice versa. This is not an "either/or" choice between the sacred and the scientific but instead incorporates a "both/and" understanding. Yes, what pastoral care is about does involve something of the sacred and the mystery *and yet* it can be investigated, defined and, in some instances, measured. The two do not cancel each other out.

SCIENCE, HEALTH CARE AND THEOLOGY

One of the earliest discoveries I made in my CPE residency was that medicine is not as absolute a science as generally believed. When first confronted with a patient situation where the difficulty was in finding the diagnosis a physician explained to me how a diagnosis is determined. The phrase she used which was a news flash for my naiveté was "medical diagnosis is really an educated guess." That was certainly not the way I had previously understood medical care. From childhood onward I had been introduced and indoctrinated in the idea that physicians knew absolutely everything with certainty, comparable almost to the divine. I believe popular vernacular would indicate that MD stands for "medical deity" in the majority of human minds.

Certainly there are scientific facts about how particular antibiotics, treatments, surgery, etc., respond to and intervene in the disease process. And these facts are utilized in the process of making a diagnosis. The physician who explained diagnosis to me said that any diagnosis is theoretically a process of detecting which symptoms correlate with a particular disease as defined by knowing which diseases are usually found in light of those particular symptoms. I began to understand that a physician looks at all the symptoms and then, for all practical purposes, makes an educated guess. Some physicians are particularly good and, indeed, may be better than others in their diagnostic talent. Sometimes diagnosis is difficult because it requires a lengthy and complex process of elimination.

A simple example occurs when a person exhibits a sore and reddened throat and an elevated temperature. A doctor, consulting his or her years of practice and knowledge, makes the educated guess that a person has strep throat and proceeds to have a culture done to prove the hypothesis. If the culture comes back negative for strep, then the doctor again reviews the symptoms and proposes another possible scenario–perhaps a sinus infection due to excess nasal drainage. This, the physician described to me, is what constitutes the ability to diagnose as an educated guess.

In a similar, but not identical vein, haven't biblical scholars used the "educated guess" in determining the origin of biblical literature? Were there not some "scientific hypothesis" suggested regarding the dates of events in the New and Old Testament? Isn't the delving into what is known as the "Q source" a scientific endeavor to determine, with the best educated guess, when the earliest written text was recorded? Using a set of methods used to determine and measure authenticity, dates, context and possible meaning found in the texts, scholars can hypothesize and generate theories, but they cannot prove with absolute certainty that they are right. A scientific method does not guarantee certainty, neither in medicine nor exegesis.

WILL DEFINING AND MEASURING THE DISCIPLINE DILUTE THE ART?

This question makes the implication that, until recently, the activity of defining and measuring the discipline of pastoral care hasn't existed. And according to scientific standards the statement is accurate. The current wave of research is not focusing on pastoral care per se. Rather the research is being done to understand the effect a spiritual or religious practice might have on illness. (The issue and debate between what is pastoral care as opposed to spiritual care is a whole other topic albeit related.) I would add here that in making a positive correlation between spiritual practices and health the implication *may not necessarily* be a bonus for pastoral care providers.

One of the obvious problems has to do with the fact that professional pastoral care providers have not written the books, produced the research or created the publicity that would address the definition and the practice of pastoral care. Otherwise, the question of "What is a chaplain? would cease to occur in hospital settings with regularity. The knowledge of what a chaplain does can be equally lacking. I would suspect that in the younger generations this would be even more so. At least our generation has a clue with Fr. Mulcahy of "Mash" fame. How many laments have I heard that with all of the hospital and medical TV shows that exist only on a rare occasion do we see a chaplain.

The fact that we have not done a better job in presenting our work is not solely due to a lack of research. There is, however, an obvious gap somewhere along the way if the current climate would have us believe that the link between religion and health is a major discovery.

Has our silence been a result that we are unable to speak clearly about what we do and how we do it, perhaps reflecting a lack of authority? Or, is our silence due to the belief that pastoral care and ministry are sacred tasks beyond reach of definition, perhaps reflecting too much authority? Are we arrogant or inept?

There is the fact that for many years pastoral care has co-opted the language of psychology when faced with the dilemma of needing to find a place among the disciplines. We are thankful that through much recent work, beginning with Paul Pruyser's *Minister as Diagnostician* (1996), we have begun to claim our own language as a basis for pastoral assessment and intervention. And although many have done outstanding work in beginning this process, there still is a measure of resistance when the call goes out to chaplains that they do need to do research. Some chaplains have urged us to give attention to research for years and I am certainly one of the resistant ones.

The actual content of pastoral care may vary in accordance with a particular faith tradition but there is an ability to describe the practice of professional pastoral care. There is a body of knowledge about the tasks of guiding, healing, and sustaining those who are hurting souls, i.e., pastoral theology. The practice involves theologically educated persons who are clinically trained in the application of his or her tradition to provide care. The particulars of the care are within the framework of faith and yet able to converse and counsel with persons from all traditions or those who lack any tradition. The care involves understanding a person's framework for viewing the world, others around them and the ability to look beyond to a transcending or transforming of life's experiences. This care most often provides the patient, family or staff within an institution the increased ability to utilize hope, comfort, and challenge. The outcome *may* be an enhanced understanding and acceptance of situations that are dis-eased and distressing. There may be an increased ability to utilize the hope, comfort and challenge as a means to cope with a newly diagnosed chronic illness, which has altered a way of life for someone. There may be a decrease in anxiety both physical and spiritual. At the least, sound pastoral care can provide a person with an opportunity to create meaning in a situation that is interpreted as meaningless. This is certainly true in the midst of intense grief and despair. Even the temporary measures of comfort and consolation given in an emergency trauma situation are often remembered and described as incredibly helpful and sustaining.

The specific tasks of providing this care are numerous. Chaplains have the skills of listening and sorting through the person's words or actions apart from his or her projections. They are trained to know when and how a particular intervention or response might be helpful, i.e., the difference between an open-ended question and a confirming statement. Chaplains have the ability to hear confessions, deep concerns and laments in such a way that a person experiences a degree of confidence and/or grace. Often the patient can be helped to have a greater sense of self and self-control in a situation in which by definition there is lack or loss of control (i.e., disease). Furthermore, the chaplain represents a community, which offers an environment of support and reconciliation.

The result of these interventions has the possibility to relieve a person who is experiencing spiritual pain. The effects of this relief are the current focus of attention within research. The outcomes of how an intervention of this type contributes to an overall sense of health and well being are being measured.

Finally, in line with the first section of my response I would propose the following. If the critical methodologies used to understand the sacred texts have, in fact, created a deeper sense of meaning and understanding of the faith, then would it not have the same potential within the field of professional chaplaincy and pastoral care? My answer would be a resounding yes but with the understanding that scientific study alone is not a panacea.

THE FINAL ANSWER

The third theme in my response follows the initial ambivalence, which began these thoughts. The question of whether professional chaplaincy and pastoral education should become more scientific in response to health care reform cannot be answered with a simple yes or no. That is clearly an unnecessary dualistic approach.

I believe that most of us engaged in the practice and teaching of pastoral care are not on a particular "side" of this debate. The sides presented, however, do characterize the variety of views within professional chaplaincy as we wrestle with a changing health care world. The current avalanche of research is painfully absent of the voice from pastoral care.

And if we can challenge ourselves to examine the lack of a voice in order that our thinking and energy are stimulated than perhaps there will not be such silence. We might even take a direction that is characterized as an attempt to evangelize. Acknowledging that becoming more scientific is only a *means to the end* can do this. The end, I would propose, is to proclaim that there is meaning to be found within religious faith. And when we are able to find a way to practice our faith in a healthy manner we ultimately manifest the Divine and the Holy Other.

REFERENCE

Pruyser, P. (1976). *The Minister as Diagnostician*. Phil: The Westminster Press.

Index

Access-related issues
  access *vs.* equity, 204-208
  needs-access considerations, 116
Accountability, professional
  Association for Clinical Pastoral
    Education (ACPE) and, 117,
    121-123
  Clinical Pastoral Education (CPE)
    and, 121-123
  contexts of, 115-117
    accrediting agencies and, 115
    alternative and complementary
      therapies and, 115
    cultural interests and, 115-116
    economic considerations and,
      116
    ethical perspectives and, 117
    introduction to, 115
    needs-access considerations of,
      116
    spirituality definitions and,
      116-117
    technology-related issues, 116
  distinguishing marks of, 118-121
  future perspectives of, 122-123
  historical perspectives of, 115-117
  internal *vs.* external work and, 118
  introduction to, 113-115
  outcome measures and, 118-120
  reference and research literature
    about, 123
  training- and education-related
    issues of, 121-123
Accrediting agencies, 115
Action directions, 108-111
Administrative-related perspectives
  Clinical Pastoral Education (CPE)
    and, 166

education theory and practice and,
  167-168
future perspectives of, 170
health care reform and, 169-170
introduction to, 165-167
post-critical world views, 170
provider-results orientations, 168
research categorization, 167-168
Allport, G. W., 103-104,215-218
Alternative and complementary
  therapies, 115
Ambiguity *vs.* security, 207-208
Art *vs.* science tensions, 144-145
Assessments, spiritual, 47,239-240
Association for Clinical Pastoral
  Education (ACPE)
  Emmanuel Movement and, 100-102
  integrated-related approaches and,
    147
  professional accountability and,
    117,121-123
  research processes and, 96
  research-informed approaches and,
    68,70
  science-religion similarities and, 30,
    37-38
  training-related perspectives and,
    237
Association of Professional Chaplains
  (APC), 68-71
Augsberger, D., 231-234

Bacon, F., 33
Baroody, J., 1-10
Baugh, W. J., 11-17
Bay, P. S., 19-27
Best practices, 23-24

Bioethical decision-making, 52-62
Bly, R., 20
Boggle factor, 85-86
Boisen, A., 1-10,21,39,126
Brown, W. N., 29-41
Burton, L., 43-51
Business models, 24

Care, pastoral *vs.* nursing, 239-240
Carey, L. B., 53-65
Categorization, research, 167-168
Circle of influence frameworks,
     205-206
Classification schema, 215
Client-centered *vs.* psychoanalytic
     orientations, 214-215
Clinical Pastoral Education (CPE) and
     research. *See also* under
     individual topics
administrative-related perspectives
     of, 166
empirical research perspectives of,
     53-64
evidence-based chaplaincy and, 191
health care reform and, 152-155
historical perspectives of, xiii-xiv,
     1-10
   Boisen, A. and, 1,3-6
   future perspectives of, 10
   importance of, 7-10
   introduction to, xiii-xiv,1-3
   reference and research literature
        about, 10
   Worcester, E. and, 1,3-6
integrated-related approaches to,
     147
introduction to, xiii-xviii
investment-related approaches to,
     105
outcome measures and, 12
phenomenological research model
     and, 171-183
philosophical approaches and,
     214-215,219-220

professional accountability and,
     121-123
reference and research literature
     about, xiv
research processes and, 93-96
research-informed approaches to,
     70-71
responses to, xvii-xviii
science-religion similarities and,
     37-39
synthesis-related perspectives of,
     131-133,137-140
systems theory approaches to, 20,
     23-27
training-related perspectives of,
     69-71,238,240-241
Coaching, employee, 105-106
Collaboration-related issues, 87,99
COMISS initiatives, 154
Communications skills, interpersonal,
     126
Compassion *vs.* science, 23-24
Complementary and alternative
     therapies, 115
Conflict models, 106-107
Contexts, professional accountability,
     115-117
Convergences
   faith-health, 100-101
   religion-science, 188-189
Copernicus, xiii
Coping methods, 190-191
Cost-effective modalities, 21-22
Critical evaluations, 55-56
Critical methodologies, 243
Critiques, research, 13-14
Croteau, J., 179-183
Cultural interests, 115-116
Cures *vs.* healings, 136

De Chardin, T., 29,33-35,40
Decision-making processes
   bioethics and, 52-62
   outcome measures and, 14-15

Directions
    action, 108-111
    research, 81-89. *See also* Research
        Directions
Discipline definitions, 241-243
Dualistic approaches, 243-244
Dykstra, C., 20,25
Dynamic processes, 22
Dysfunctional systems, 21

Economic reform, 108,116
Education- and training-related issues
    Clinical Pastoral Education (CPE).
        See Clinical Pastoral
        Education (CPE) and
        research
    description of, 69-71
    education theory and practice,
        167-168
    process education model, 93
Effectiveness-related issues, 69,94-95,
        135-140
Efficacy-related issues, 101-102
Einstein, A., 32,195
Elijah, 189
Emmanuel Movement
    Association for Clinical Pastoral
        Education (ACPE) and,
        100-102
    Clinical Pastoral Education (CPE)
        and, 99-102
    collaborations and, 99
    efficacy-related issues of, 101-102
    faith-health convergences and,
        100-101
    future perspectives of, 101-102
    identity-related perspectives of,
        101-102
    introduction to, 99-100
    lines of responsibility, blurring of,
        99-100
    moral urgency and, 100
    reference and research literature
        about, 102

Empirical research perspectives
    in Australia and New Zealand,
        53-64
    bioethical decision-making and,
        52-62
    Clinical Pastoral Education (CPE)
        and, 53-64
    critical evaluations and, 55-56
        introduction to, 55
        methods of, 56
        research training, lack of, 55-56
        student-centered learning and, 55
    empiricism and, 85
    future perspectives of, 62-64
    introduction to, 53-55
    reference and research literature
        about, 64-65
    research levels and, 53-62
        introduction to, 53-56
        macro-level, 60-62
        meso-level, 59-60
        micro-level, 56-59
Employee coaching, 105-106
Equity *vs.* access, 204-208
Erickson, M., 32-33
Ethical perspectives, 117
Evaluations, critical, 55-56
Evidence-based chaplaincy
    future perspectives of, 191-192
    introduction to, 185-186
    reference and research literature
        about, 192-194
    religion-science convergences and,
        188-189
        introduction to, 188
        patient spirituality and, 188-189
        religion-science integration and,
            189
        truth-seeking roles and, 188
        universe origin-seeking roles
            and, 188
    spiritual leadership roles and,
        190-191
        Clinical Pastoral Education
            (CPE) and, 191

coping methods and, 190-191
    introduction to, 190
vs. evidence-based health care,
    186-188
    introduction to, 186
    patient-provider relationships
        and, 187
    published research roles and,
        186-187
    qualitative research roles and,
        187
vs. tradition-driven chaplaincy,
    189-190
    clinical methods and, 190
    faith *vs.* evidence and, 189
    historical perspectives of, 190
    introduction to, 189
Evidence-based health care, 186-188
Existential phenomenology model,
    180-183
Existentialism, 230
Expanded science development,
    227-228
Experiential knowledge, 24
External *vs.* internal work, 118

Fads, theological, 9
Faith-health convergences, 100-101
Fear-related issues, 44
Fitchett, G., 67-79
Flaws, spirituality research
    generational differences and,
        125-126
    interpersonal communications skills
        and, 126
    introduction to, 125-130
    presumptions and, 127-130
        God, scientific research of,
            127-128
        historical-political entities,
            spirituality of, 128-129
        multiculturalism and, 128-129
        prayer, research about, 129-130
        religion, effectiveness of, 130

spirituality, as one entity, 127
        value sets and, 129-130
    religion *vs.* art and, 125-126
    scientific *vs.* spiritual flaws and,
        130
    truth, scientific assessments of, 126
Focus, professional, 16-17
FOCUS-PDCA model, 200-201,
    204-205
FOCUS-PDSA model, 200-201,
    204-205
Four compass points, health care
    reform, 198-208
Frameworks, circle of influence,
    205-206
Freud, S., xiv,2
Future perspectives
    of administrative-related
        perspectives, 170
    of the Emmanuel Movement,
        101-102
    of empirical research perspectives,
        62-64
    of evidence-based chaplaincy,
        191-192
    of health care reform, 160-161,
        208-210
    of historical perspectives, 10
    of identity-related perspectives,
        49-50
    of integrated-related approaches,
        144
    of investment-related approaches,
        111
    of narrative-based perspectives,
        235-236
    of outcome measures, 16-17
    of the phenomenological research
        model, 182-183
    of philosophical approaches,
        219-220
    of professional accountability,
        122-123
    of research directions, 88-89
    of research processes, 96-97

of research-informed approaches,
78-79
of science-religion similarities,
38-39
of synthesis-related perspectives,
139-140
of systems theory approaches, 27
of training-related perspectives,
243-244

Gadamer, H. G., 231-234
Galileo, xiii
Generational differences, 125-126
God, scientific research of, 127-128
Grigori, A., 179-180

Hammerskjold, D., 34
Healing environment creation, 25-26
Healings *vs.* cures, 136
Health care reform
administrative-related perspectives
of, 169-170
Clinical Pastoral Education (CPE)
and, 152-155
four compass points of, 198-208
access *vs.* equity, 204-208
circle of influence framework
and, 205-206
introduction to, 198
legislative *vs.* economic
pressures, 202-204
quality control *vs.* process
improvement, 198-201
technology-related issues, 201-202
future perspectives of, 160-161,
208-210
historical perspectives of, 197-198
integrated disciplines and, 199-200
integrated-related approaches to,
147-150
interaction to, 151-152,195-197
limitations of, 198

as misbegotten notion, 152-161
models for, 200-205
FOCUS-PDCA,
200-201,204-205
FOCUS-PDSA,
200-201,204-205
illness, 207-208
SWOT (strengths-weaknesses-
opportunities-threats),
200-201
reference and research literature
about, 162-163,210-211
resistance-related issues of,
157-158
resource-related issues of, 153-154
responses to, positive *vs.* negative,
xv-xviii
scientific meanings and, 154-156
security *vs.* ambiguity and, 207-208
service-related issues of, 158-160
systems processes and, 206-207
Hidden spiritual dynamics, 235-236
Hilsman, G. J., 81-89
Historical perspectives
of Association for Clinical Pastoral
Education (ACPE), 6
Boisen, A. and, 1-10
of Clinical Pastoral Education
(CPE), 1-10
future perspectives of, 10
importance of, 7-10
introduction to, xiii-xiv,1-3
of philosophical approaches,
213-218
of professional accountability,
115-117
of pseudo-faith, 10
reference and research literature
about, 10
of scientific faith, 9-10
of theological fads, 9
of tradition-driven chaplaincy, 190
Worcester, E. and, 1,3-6
Historical-political entities, spirituality
of, 128-129

Holistic health, 135-136
Hover, M., 91-97
Huffstutler, E. W., 99-102

Identity-related perspectives
  controversial issues of, 45-46
  of the Emmanuel Movement,
    101-102
  fear-related issues of, 44,46-47
  future perspectives of, 49-50
  introduction to, 43-44
  moral obligation-related issues of,
    48-49
  performance improvement-related
    issues of, 48-49
  reference and research literature
    about, 50-51
  research criteria and, 45
  role-related issues of, 46-47,48
  self-deception and, 49
  spiritual assessments and, 47
Illness model, 207-208
Imagination, 32-33
Institutional review boards (IRBs),
  94-95
Integrated-related approaches
  art vs. science tensions and,
    144-145
  Association for Clinical Pastoral
    Education (ACPE) and, 147
  Clinical Pastoral Education (CPE)
    and, 147
  future perspectives of, 144
  health care reform and, 147-150
  integrated disciplines and, 199-200
  introduction to, 143-144
  justification-related issues of,
    146-147
  outcome measures and, 145-146
  reference and research literature
    about, 144
Integration
  integration-related approaches,
    145-146

psychological-spiritual integrative
    points, 177-180
  religion-science, 189
  vs. measurement, 87-88
Internal *vs.* external work, 118
Interpersonal communications skills, 126
Investment-related approaches
  action directions and, 108-111
  Allport, G., 103-104
  Clinical Pastoral Education (CPE)
    and, 105
  conflict models and, 106-107
  economic reform and, 108
  employee coaching and, 105-106
  future perspectives of, 111
  health care reform and, 104-105
  introduction to, 103-104
  James, W. and, 103-104
  reference and research literature
    about, 111-112
  science philosophy and, 106-107
  scientific materialism and, 106-107
Ivy, S. S., 103-112

James, W., 103-104,220,227-228
Jensen, M. E., 113-123
Jesus Christ, 7,133,140,189,207
John of the Cross (Sister), 97
John XXIII (Pope), 128
Jung, Carl, 38-39
Justification-related issues, 146-147

Knowledge, experiential, 24
Kuhn, T., 35-36, 40

Lawrence, R. J., 125-130
Leadership-related issues, 88
Leliaert, R., 131-141
Levels, research, 53-62
Lines of responsibility, blurring of,
  99-100

Literacy, research, 69
Location-specific issues, 214-215
Long obedience concept, 25-27
Lucas, A. M., 143-150

Macro-level research, 60-62
Mary Joseph (Mother), 97
Maslow, A., 227-228
Materialism, scientific, 106-107
McCurdy, D. B., 151-163
Measurability concepts, 21
Measures, outcome. *See* Outcome
    measures
Meditation, 35-36
Meso-level research, 59-60
Micro-level research, 56-59
Millspaugh, D., 165-183
Models
    business, 24
    conflict, 106-107
    education process, 93
    existential phenomenology,
        180-183
    FOCUS-PDCA, 200-201,204-205
    FOCUS-PDSA, 200-201,204-205
    illness, 207-208
    phenomenological research. *See*
        Phenomenological research
        model
    process education, 93
    SWOT (strengths-weaknesses-
        opportunities-threats),
        200-201
Modernism, psychological, 226-227
Moral obligation-related issues, 48-49
Moral urgency, 100
Moses, 13
Multiculturalism, 128-129

Narrative-based perspectives
    future perspectives of, 235-236
    introduction to, 223-225

reference and research literature
    about, 236
science and, 223-228
    expanded science development,
        227-228
    introduction to, 223-224
    psychological modernism and,
        226-227
    vs. chaplaincy, 225
    vs. theology, 225
story bearer and sharer roles,
    228-236
    Augsberger, D. and, 231-234
    definition of, 228-229
    existential and spiritual
        dimensions of, 230
    Gadamer, H. G. and, 231-234
    hidden spiritual dynamics and,
        235-236
    introduction to, 228
    listening and, 231
    professional chaplaincy and, 230
    research and, 234-235
    sadness and depression and,
        231-234
    seriousness of, 228-230
    therapeutic understanding and,
        234
    world recreation and, 231
National Association of Catholic
    Chaplains (NACC), 68
National Association of Jewish
    Chaplains (NAJC), 68
National Institute for Health Care
    Research, 154
Needs-access considerations, 116
Newell, C., 53-65
Nursing care *vs.* pastoral care, 239-240

O'Connor, T. S., 185-194
Osler, W., 23
Outcome measures
    Clinical Pastoral Education (CPE)
        and, 12

decision-making processes and,
14-15
future perspectives of, 16-17
integration-related approaches to,
145-146
introduction to, 11
measurability concepts and, 21
measurements *vs.* integration and, 87-88
paradigm shifts and, 11-17
professional accountability and,
118-120
professional focus and, 16-17
reference and research literature
about, 17
research critiques and, 13-14
research methodology and, 16-17
research processes and, 95-96
training-related perspectives of,
241-243
value justification and, 14-15

Paradigm shifts, 11-17
Pastoral care *vs.* nursing care, 239-240
Patient spirituality, 188-189
Patient-provider relationships, 187
Performance improvement-related
issues, 48-49
Phenomenological research model
chaplains as scientists and, 173-174
Clinical Pastoral Education (CPE)
and, 171-183
contemporary society and, 175-176
Croteau, J. and, 179-183
existential phenomenology model
and, 180-183
future perspectives of, 182-183
Grigori, A., 179-183
integrative points,
psychological-spiritual,
177-180
introduction to, 171-173
reality measures and, 173-174
reference and research literature
about, 183

research approaches, spiritual *vs.*
natural science, 174-175
transcendency and, 172-173
Philosophical approaches
Allport, G. W. and, 215-218
chaplaincy and, 219-220
Clinical Pastoral Education (CPE)
and, 214-215,219-220
future perspectives of, 219-220
historical perspectives of, 213-218
introduction to, 213-215
location-specific issues of, 214-215
psychoanalytic *vs.* client-centered
orientations, 214-215
reference and research literature
about, 220-221
religion and, 218-219
definitions of, 218
introduction to, 218
quantitative research and, 219
scientism and, 218-219
science and, 215-218
classification schema for, 215
dominant world views and,
216-217
introduction to, 215
roles of, 216-217
technology-related issue of,
216-217
theological and ethical education
and, 217-218
Pius IX (Pope), 129
Pius XII (Pope), 126,128-129
Polayni, M., 107
Political-historical entities, spirituality
of, 128-129
Positivism, 235-236
Post-critical world views, 170
Power-related issues, 25-26
Pragmatism, 85
Prayer
effectiveness of, 135-140
processes of, 93
research studies of, 93,129-130
Presumption-related issues, 127-130

Primacy, spiritual, 138-139
Processes
    dynamic, 22
    process education model, 93
    process improvement *vs.* quality
        control, 198-201
    research, 91-97. *See also* Research
        processes
Professionalism
    accountability and, 113-123. *See
        also* Accountability,
        professional
    professional focus, 16-17
    professional identity-related
        perspectives of, 43-51. *See
        also* Identity-related
        perspectives
    synthesis-related perspectives of,
        137-138
Provider-related issues
    patient-provider relationships, 187
    results-provider orientations, 168
Pseudo-faith, 10
Psychoanalytic *vs.* client-centered
        orientations, 214-215
Psychodynamic theory, 100
Psychological modernism, 226-227
Published research roles, 186-187

Qualitative research
    qualitative-quantitative research
        tensions, 132-133
    roles of, 187
Quality control *vs.* process
        improvement, 198-201
Quality of care, 87

Reality measures, 173-174
Reference and research literature
    about the Emmanuel Movement, 102
    about empirical research
        perspectives, 64-65
    about evidence-based chaplaincy,
        192-194
    about health care reform, 162-163,
        210-211
    about historical perspectives, 10
    about identity-related perspectives,
        50-51
    about integrated-related approaches,
        144
    about investment-related
        approaches, 111-112
    about narrative-based perspectives,
        236
    about outcome measures, 17
    about the phenomenological
        research model, 183
    about philosophical approaches,
        220-221
    about professional accountability,
        123
    about research directions, 89
    about research processes, 97
    about research-informed
        approaches, 71-72
    about science-religion similarities,
        39-41
    about synthesis-related
        perspectives, 140-141
    about systems theory approaches,
        27
    about training-related perspectives,
        244
Religion-science similarities, 29-41,
        188-189. *See also*
        Science-religion similarities
Reluctance-related issues, 37-39
Research categorization, 167-168
Research critiques, 13-14
Research directions
    boggle factor and, 85-86
    boundaries of, 86-88
        collaboration, 87
        integration *vs.* measurement,
            87-88
        introduction to, 86

leadership-related issues, 88
limitations, 88
quality of care, 87
study selection, 86-87
conjectures about, 82-84
dilemmas about, 84-85
future perspectives of, 88-89
historical perspectives of, 82-84
introduction to, 81-82
reference and research literature
about, 89
research processes and, 95-96
Research levels, 53-62
macro-level, 60-62
meso-level, 59-60
micro-level, 56-59
Research literacy, 69
Research processes
Association for Clinical Pastoral
Education (ACPE) and, 96
Clinical Pastoral Education (CPE)
and, 93-96
effectiveness-related issues of,
94-95
future perspectives of, 96-97
introduction to, 91-92
outcome measures and, 95-96
practices issues and, 95-97
prayer studies and, 93
process education model and, 93
reference and research literature
about, 97
research direction and, 95-96
scientific investigation, 93
witness-related issues and, 97
Research-informed approaches
Association for Clinical Pastoral
Education (ACPE) and, 68,
70
Association of Professional
Chaplains (APC) and, 68-71
Clinical Pastoral Education (CPE)
and, 70-71
future perspectives of, 78-79
goals of, 68-71

education and training and,
69-71
implementation of, 69-70
introduction to, 68-69
ministry effectiveness, 69
publications and, 70-71
research literacy, 69
research pursuit, 69
research value, 69
introduction to, 67-68
National Association of Catholic
Chaplains (NACC) and, 68
National Association of Jewish
Chaplains (NAJC) and, 68
rational for, 68
reference and research literature
about, 71-72
Resistance-related issues, 157-158
Resource-related issues, 153-154
Rodrigues, B., 195-211
Rogers, C., xiv,38-39
Role-related issues, 46-47,48
Rosetti, C., 197
Russell, B., 31-32

Sacks, O., 228-229
Schleiermercher, F., 31
Science philosophy, 106-107
Science vs. art tensions, 144-145
Science-religion similarities
Association for Clinical Pastoral
Education (ACPE) and, 30,
37-38
Bacon, F. and, 33
Clinical Pastoral Education (CPE)
and, 37-39
De Chardin, T. and, 29,33-35,40
Einstein, A. and, 32
Erickson, M. and, 32-33
future perspectives of, 38-39
Hammerskjold, D. and, 34
imagination and, 32-33
introduction to, 29-30
Jung, C. and, 38-39

Kuhn, T. and, 35-36,40
Mach, E. and, 31
meditation and, 35-36
in practice, 33-34
reference and research literature
    about, 39-41
religion-science convergences and,
    188-189
reluctance-related issues of, 37-39
Rogers, C. and, 38-39
Russell, B. and, 31-32
Schleiermercher, F. and, 31
science as art and, 36-37
scientific methods and, 34-36
vs. science-religion separation,
    30-32
Wilber, K. and, 34-35
Scientific faith, 9-10
Scientific materialism, 106-107
Scientism, 218-219
Security *vs.* ambiguity, 207-208
Self-deception, 49
Seltzer, R., 228
Separation, science-religion, 30-32
Service-related issues, 158-160
Shakespeare, W., 96-97
Similarities, science-religion, 29-41.
    See also Science-religion
    similarities
Spiritual assessments, 47,239-240
Spiritual leadership roles, 190-191
Spiritual primacy, 138-139
Spiritual research. *See* Clinical
    Pastoral Education (CPE) and
    research
Story bearer and sharer roles, 228-236
Strunk, O. C., 213-221
Student-centered learning, 55
Swinton, J., 223-236
SWOT (strengths-weaknesses-
    opportunities-threats) model,
    200-201
Synthesis-related perspectives
    Clinical Pastoral Education (CPE)
        and, 131-140

cures *vs.* healings and, 136
future perspectives of, 139-140
holistic health and, 135-136
introduction to, 131-133
prayer effectiveness and, 135-140
professionalism and, 137-138
qualitative-quantitative research
    tensions, 132-133
reference and research literature
    about, 140-141
scientific limitations and, 136
spiritual primacy and, 138-139
Systems processes, 206-207
Systems theory approaches
    best practices and, 23-24
    business models and, 24
    Clinical Pastoral Education (CPE)
        and, 20,23-27
    compassion *vs.* science and, 23-24
    cost-effective modalities and, 21-22
    dynamic processes and, 22
    dysfunctional systems and, 21
    experiential knowledge and, 24
    future perspectives of, 27
    healing environment creation and,
        25-26
    health care contexts and, 22
    introduction to, 19-20
    long obedience concept and, 25-27
    measurability concepts and, 21
    power-related issues and, 25-26
    reference and research literature
        about, 27
    systems processes and, 206-207

Technology-related issues, 116,
    201-202,216-217
Tertullian, xiii
Theological fads, 9
Therapeutic understanding, 234
Thomas (Apostle), 189
Tradition-driven chaplaincy, 189-190
Training-related perspectives

Association for Clinical Pastoral
    Education (ACPE) and, 237
Clinical Pastoral Education (CPE)
    and, 69-71,238,240-241
critical methodologies and, 243
discipline definitions and, 241-243
dualistic approaches and, 243-244
future perspectives of, 243-244
introduction to, 69-71,237-238
outcome measures and, 241-243
pastoral care *vs.* nursing care,
    239-240
reference and research literature
    about, 244
science-health care-theology
    relationships, 240-241
spiritual assessments and, 239-240
Transcendency, 172-173
Truth
    scientific assessments of, 126
    truth-seeking roles, 188

Universe origin-seeking roles, 188
Urgency, moral, 100

Value-related issues
    research, value of, 69
    value justification, 14-15
    value sets, 129-130
VandeCreek, L., xiii-xviii

Wilber, K., 27,34-35
Wilson, J. C., 237-244
Witness-related issues, 97
Worcester, E., 1,3-6
Work, internal *vs.* external, 118
World recreation, 231

Zeitgeist, 213,219-220

Professional Chaplaincy and Clinical Pastoral Education Should Become More Scientific

Yes and No

___ in softbound at $18.71 (regularly $24.95) (ISBN: 0-7890-2238-9)
___ in hardbound at $26.21 (regularly $34.95) (ISBN: 0-7890-2237-0)